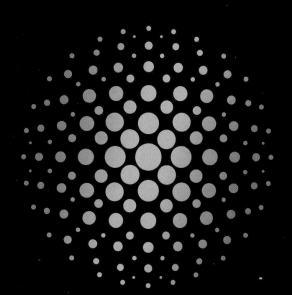

QUANTUMYOGA®

CREATING YOUR **IDEAL PRACTICE** FROM AN OCEAN OF POSSIBILITIES

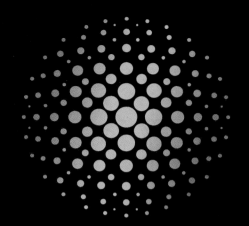

QUANTUMYOGA®

CREATING YOUR **IDEAL PRACTICE** FROM AN OCEAN OF POSSIBILITIES

LARA BAUMANN

MANDALA
PUBLISHING

MANDALA
PUBLISHING

Mandala Publishing
3160 Kerner Blvd. Unit 108
San Rafael. CA 94901
www.mandala.org
800.668.2218

Library of Congress Cataloging–in–Publication Data available

ISBN-13: 978-1601090188
ISBN-10: 1601090188

  REPLANTED PAPER

ROOTS of PEACE

Palace Press International, in association with Roots of Peace,
will plant two trees for each tree used in the manufacturing of this
book. Roots of Peace is an internationally renowned humanitarian
organization dedicated to eradicating land mines worldwide and
converting war-torn lands into productive farms and wildlife
habitats. Together, we will plant two million fruit and nut trees in
Afghanistan and provide farmers there with the skills and support
necessary for sustainable land use.

PALACE PRESS
INTERNATIONAL

Printed in China by Palace Press International
www.palacepress.com

The content of this book is provided for informational purposes
only, and is not intended to diagnose, treat, or cure any
conditions without the assistance of a trained practitioner.
If you are experiencing any medical condition, seek care
from an appropriate licensed professional.

www.quantumyoga.co.uk

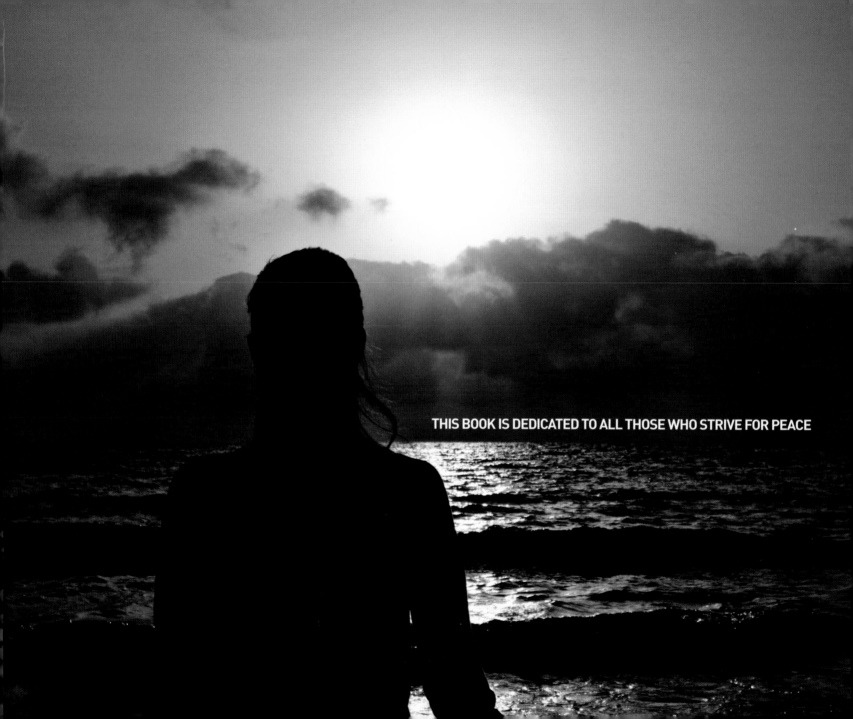

THIS BOOK IS DEDICATED TO ALL THOSE WHO STRIVE FOR PEACE

INTRODUCTION

Q uantum Yoga developed organically from my own yoga practice, in an endeavor to bring together the various styles and philosophies I have studied and extract their essence, to find an accessible and universal application. My aim was to create a harmonious flow that would leave the body strong, the mind still, the emotions steady, and the heart open and joyful. In the beginning I practiced totally freestyle, but soon realized that on most days this was not satisfactory and that I needed a systematic framework around which to design. I found that a framework actually stimulates, rather than restricts, creativity and leaves room for spontaneous variation and intuitive response. Furthermore, the microcosm of the body changes as consciousness spreads through it, and therefore *asana* practice becomes a disciplined yet evolving communication with the body-mind. The greatest challenge is to keep up this level of awareness while allowing for playful creativity. If you don't enjoy something, you are not going to keep doing it. Make sure therefore to develop a practice that will be a faithful companion for the rest of your life! This book is designed to help you do so.

The Quantum Method of Yoga is constructed in two parts. Part one, which may be skipped by those eager to start practicing, provides the background information you'll need to understand the meaning of yoga, its history, and the way various traditions realize the ultimate goal of union with the

divine ground of being. It is important to recognize that there are many ways to attain an enlightened state of consciousness, and no one book would be able to initiate you into it all. Nevertheless, we cannot get around the body, as this is the sanctum we inhabit.

As this is primarily a book that prepares you for asana, *pranayama*, and meditation practice, the focus is on the influences that have informed this particular path to self-realization. Among the influences explained and integrated in the pages that follow are the principles of *Ayurveda*, the medical and healing branch of Vedic science, an understanding of which can support your assessment of an ideal self-practice. Also presented are other yoga paths, such as devotion, charitable acts, and study of the ancient scriptures, as well as yogic methods using music and visual cosmic diagrams. Correlations between these and asana practice show you how to put them to practical use. Lastly, I discuss a few basic insights of quantum physics, and how these can inform the way we approach spiritual practice.

Part two is devoted to individualizing the yoga practice and designed to refine the relationship with the body-heart-mind complex through which we experience life. Quantum Yoga encourages us to honor our unique requirements, and by providing a framework within which to do so, allows us to respond creatively to the messages we are being sent. In this way, yoga practice can become a steady and joyful love affair with that part of us which we will soon come to recognize as divine. Once we cultivate this experience within, we will gain the power to consciously transform the reality around us, not by manipulating it to serve our needs and ambitions, but by inspiring it to vibrate at the frequency of loving awareness.

First, the Quantum Assessment Methods are described. The choosing of a theme and a peak pose is explained, as well as how to sustain the flow and link the asana in novel ways. Next, the Quantum Grouping and Sequencing Laws are fully outlined, with photos and detailed descriptions. The three Basic Quantum Sequences are presented in their entirety with fully illustrated charts, which serve the practitioner as sample vinyasa sequences for the regulation of each of the three Ayurvedic doshas (bodily constitutions) in turn. Additional practice of pranayama and restorative and menstrual alternatives are also presented. Finally, some inspiring practical advice on how to get started is given.

The accompanying Quantum Yoga DVD represents a launchpad towards self-practice and can either be watched as an informative guide or used as real-time instruction to be practiced alongside to. Here I teach each Basic Quantum Sequence to students who are typical for their biological constitutions, or dosha. It shows case studies in which physical and emotional impediments are integrated and overcome by embracing the Ayurvedic holistic approach of recognizing body-mind type and applying this to Quantum Yoga practice. It also includes a succinct introduction to Quantum Yoga, the presentation of a basic Menstrual Practice, a Pranayama section, and a brief explanation of the concept of drishti (one-pointed focus).

Eventually, the time will come when you can try slotting in your own variations using your understanding of the Quantum Grouping and Sequencing Laws as well as the typing of postures. Each Basic Quantum Sequence regulates a particular Ayurvedic biological humor, or dosha. Remember, however, that the doshas always exist together and that a balanced sequence must work with all three while recognizing which dosha needs the most attention and thus informs the sequence's overall mood.

In Patanjali's Yoga Sutras, he calls your attention from the start: Atha Yoga Anushashanam (I,1). Now, not later, not in theory, now as you are reading, now unfolds the practice of yoga. And the butterfly flaps its wings . . .

CONTENT

PART ONE

CHAPTER ONE THE YOGA TRADITION

THE MEANING OF YOGA	010
HISTORICAL ROOTS	014
IMPORTANT SCRIPTURES	016
MAJOR CURRENT STREAMS OF HATHA YOGA	023
YOGA AND QUANTUM PHYSICS	025
THE TRUE NATURE OF REALITY	025
THE QUANTUM METHOD OF YOGA	026
THE POWER OF MANIFESTATION	027
THE PRACTICAL RELEVANCE OF ENERGY AND MATTER	029
WHAT WE KNOW NOW IS THAT WE DON'T KNOW	030
YET WE ALWAYS KNEW . . .	031

CHAPTER TWO YOGA ANATOMY AND AYURVEDA

THE RELATIONSHIP BETWEEN GROSS AND SUBTLE ANATOMY	034
AN OVERVIEW OF SUBTLE ANATOMY IN QUANTUM YOGA PRACTICE	038
THE QUANTUM SCIENCE OF SPIRITUALITY	045
AYURVEDA: THE SCIENCE OF LIFE	047
THE QUANTUM ASSESSMENT METHODS	052

PART TWO

CHAPTER THREE THE QUANTUM YOGA GROUPING AND SEQUENCING LAWS

SUSTAINING THE FLOW AND LINKING	060
TIMINGS	060
LEADING WITH LEFT OR RIGHT	061
USE OF PROPS	061
ADJUSTMENTS	062
PAIN	063
CLASSIFICATION OF ASANA ACCORDING TO PHYSIOLOGICAL EXPRESSION AND ENERGETIC EFFECT	064
HOW OFTEN SHOULD I PRACTICE?	065
FOOD	066
THE QUALITY OF YOUR PRACTICE	066
BEAUTY AND TRUTH: "THE GOLDEN SECTION"	067

THE TEN GROUPS:	068
1) SUBLIMATIO	070
2) DYNAMIC FLOW	084
3) STANDING POSES	098
4) STANDING BALANCES AND ARM BALANCES	106
5) FLOOR WORK: FORWARD-BENDS, TWISTS, SHOULDER AND HIP-OPENERS	114
6) ABDOMINALS	128
7) BACKBENDS	132
8) INVERSIONS	138
9) RELAXATION	144
10) MEDITATION	148

CHAPTER FOUR THE THREE BASIC QUANTUM SEQUENCES

BIRDS	154
HEROES	155
LOTUS MANDALA	156
PRACTICING THE THREE BASIC QUANTUM SEQUENCES	157
THE BIRDS SEQUENCE	158
THE HEROES SEQUENCE	170
THE LOTUS MANDALA SEQUENCE	178

CHAPTER FIVE ADDITIONAL PRACTICE

PURE PRANAYAMA	192
RESTORATIVE, MENSTRUAL AND PREGNANCY QUANTUM YOGA PRACTICE	202
MUDRAS AND KRIYAS	212
SOUND, VISION AND TOUCH: FURTHER SUPPORTS FOR SELF-PRACTICE	215
CREATING YOUR IDEAL YOGA PRACTICE: GETTING STARTED	222
PERSONAL PRACTICE WORKSHEET	227

LARA BAUMANN'S YOGA BIOGRAPHY	228

Caution Practitioners should not try to complete all sequences or breathing exercises at first. If in doubt, consult your doctor before beginning this or any yoga program without the direct assistance of a qualified teacher. The following instructions are in no way intended as a substitute for medical counselling. The author disclaims any liability for injury resulting from the procedures in this book.

PART ONE

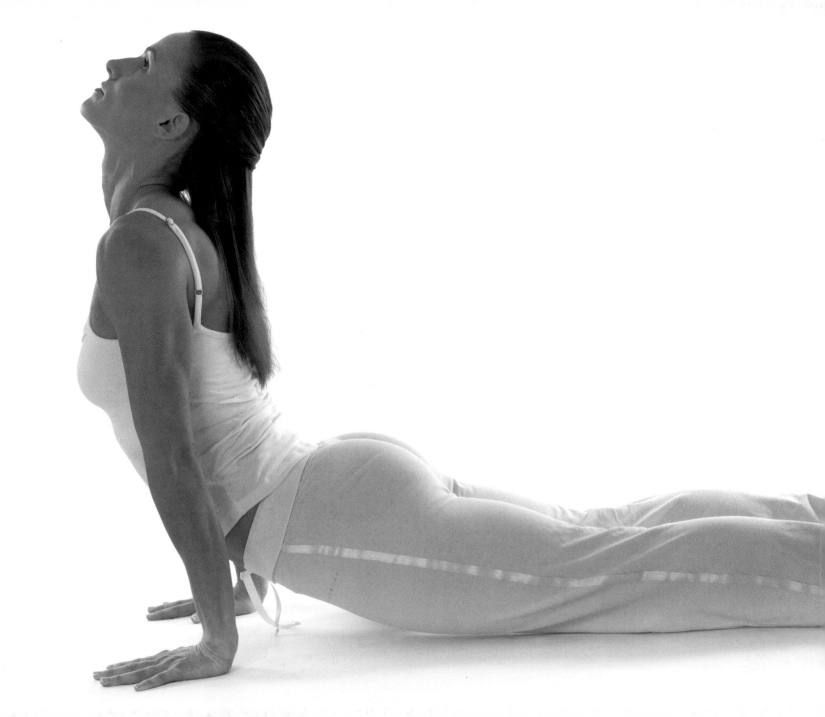

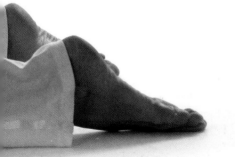

CHAPTER ONE
THE YOGA TRADITION

THE MEANING OF YOGA

Like many spiritual endeavors, one of yoga's central aims appears to be a paradox—be present in the body to get beyond the mind. A misidentification with fluctuating mind-states and the emotions they generate, as well as with the experience of an imperfect reality that is borne out of this turbulence, is recognized as the root of all the suffering we encounter. According to yogis and mystics of old, our true essence, pure consciousness, is of the nature of bliss, peace, and radiant clarity. So how do we go about stilling the mind? How do we deliberately stop the thoughts turning around in our heads and pierce through to a realization of ultimate truth?

In order to overcome something, we must know that thing. In order to truly know a thing, we have to be that thing. Thus knower and known become one and the result is knowledge revealed through pure consciousness. We already carry this wisdom, but to realize it, we must experience it. There is one way only to unlock the mechanism of revelation: practice.

Patanjali begins his Yoga Sutras with the famous definition: *Yogash Chitta Vrtti Nirodha* (I, 2) (Yoga is the cessation of the fluctuations in consciousness). "Yoga is the stopping of mental turbulence," would be another way of translating this definition. In India, sacred knowledge has been handed down in an oral tradition to the rishis, or seers, since ancient times.

Patanjali compiled much of this knowledge pertaining to yoga into 195 aphorisms called *sutras* in Sanskrit, which means "threads that bind together".

The word *yoga*, which occurs in the Rigveda, an ancient sacred collection of Sanskrit hymns, is most frequently used in the sense of "to join or yoke," like horses being yoked to a cart. Later it came to be used as "yoking the senses." The senses were viewed as wild horses that needed to be disciplined, lest they cause attachment and pain. The mind, always preoccupied with memories and projections, came to be regarded as the master sense, which only in the nondual state of complete stillness reflects ultimate truth. In the later Upanishads, *yoga* also came to mean being near your teacher and receiving spiritual instruction.

A more commonly used meaning for the word *yoga* is "union," which is drawn from later teachings that are strongly tantric in flavor. Practice using body and breath to harness and manipulate life force (prana) steps into the foreground, and the union that is talked about is that between energy (*Shakti*) and wisdom (*Shiva*). So whereas the orthodox traditions described above advocate mostly meditative disciplines, later developments embraced the ecstasy of total sense immersion in nature (Tantra Yoga), the deliverance through grace that results from devotion (Bhakti Yoga), the retributive benefits of rightful action (Karma Yoga), as well as the wisdom gained from study of the ancient scriptures (Jnana Yoga). All paths lead ultimately to a total absorption of the self in its divine essence, which has a transformative effect that leads away from ego-bound thought to an enlightened state of consciousness and hence freedom (moksha) or liberation (kaivalya).

Yoga has a threefold meaning in that it encompasses the aim, the act, and the achievement. To join (or yoke) also means to free oneself from the reign of what was previously holding one back. This is done through discipline and control. The result is freedom from the pain caused by the domination of the ego-mind, giving way to a state of union with the Absolute. This union, or yoga, manifests as peace and bliss.

Hatred, greed, delusion, and the inevitable suffering that ensues are a result of a misidentification (maya) with the impermanent and ever-changing reality we experience all around us. We seek satisfaction and gratification from the interaction of the senses with objects, and the preoccupation of the mind with a fluctuating world. We are under the illusion that objects and the qualities we attribute to them exist independently of our awareness of them, and do not realize that the mind manifests our reality. Thus our sense of self is conditioned and relies on this continuous and futile circle of bondage (samsara). It is only when the mind becomes

completely still that it reflects back the eternal divine principle of ultimate reality. If this state can be sustained, it results in a transcendental shift in consciousness that will transform the individual's life.

Yoga constitutes a set of practices that were devised in order to experience the sublime truth that lies at the foundation of our life. It is not a belief system, but a set of practices designed to give the yogi an empirical knowledge of Spirit. Ever since the human being has had the luxury to no longer be preoccupied with basic survival and thus contemplate the source of existence and the meaning of life, there has been a longing to satisfy these spiritual yearnings. Yoga grew out of this longing and thus represents a wealth of ancient practices designed to experience the divine and realize the true nature of reality. It was always clear to the sages of yoga that whatever we experience hinges on our state of mind.

Why Quantum Yoga? Quantum physics has made incredible discoveries that echo the ancient insights of yoga. Yoga implicitly recognizes that the intellect cannot grasp ultimate reality, as knowledge intrinsically implies the duality of knower and known. Yoga represents the effort, application, and the resulting state of knowing, so it is the act of practicing as well as the end result. Hence the importance of practice over speculation. Nevertheless, as most of us do function through the intellect, there is much to be gained by assimilating yoga with the insights that quantum physics offers us. The cross-pollination that has occurred in the fields of science and metaphysics in the past few years serves the individual with inspiration and empowerment.

Quantum physics has proven that energy and matter are not so easily divisible, that in fact energy is more substantial than matter itself. In yoga practice we actually experience this insight firsthand. The body is not merely flesh and bone; it is imbued with prana, life force. All mental fluctuations have a direct effect on this pranic flow, which in turn manifests as physical sensations and disease. We can revert this process by addressing body, breath, and mind in a holistic manner. To this end, we must first become conscious of the interaction of all three, which will be different in each individual. Then we should learn how to intelligently apply the ancient tools of yoga to our personal needs in such a manner that we return to our unique state of perfection.

For what is true yoga practice, if not one that awakens our capacity to hear the inner voice of wisdom? For yoga to be a transformative practice, it must take into account personal, physical, emotional, and spiritual challenges. Yoga denotes a yoking to truth and a path towards self-realization in order to attain a state of union with the Absolute. It can therefore

never be an imposition on the body-mind, but a process of communication with the higher self and a return to one's natural state of ease. Yoga is thus a shedding of sheathes, a process of purification, and an embracing of one's true nature. We are not adding anything new, but letting go of that which is not real. What we are left with is an entity whose inner radiance reflects back the divine essence that is the source of existence itself. We then recognize it in everything, and thus self-realization is nothing other than the realization of the Oneness of being.

Quantum Yoga gives the individual the tools and right knowledge (*viveka*) to spontaneously construct such an ideal practice. Truly taking into account your present state will also help take you into the now. *Santosha*, or contentment, is one of the *niyamas* (or observances, second Limb of Yoga) and indicates that you should work with what you have, rather than project what you think should be there. Quantum Yoga encourages deep listening (Nada Yoga) to the inner voice of insight, while integrating the insights gained into a system that the intellect can comprehend and apply. It strengthens the body's inherent intelligence, stimulates intuition, and awakens creativity. It puts the responsibility for health and happiness firmly into the individual's hands and thus allows each and every person to manifest strength, beauty, and joy.

The ultimate state of enlightenment, or samadhi, cannot be intellectually grasped, nor is it a guaranteed award even for the most ardent yogi. However, applying the tools of Quantum Yoga to continually cultivate the skill and discipline to live your truth (*dharma*) means opening to divine grace. Remember not to buy into the illusion that you are fighting against a life that is designed for suffering. Nature wants you to be free; she wants the you that is pure consciousness to throw off the shackles of the false ego and make the journey back to the source from whence you emanate. In this very incarnation we have been given the opportunity to make the journey back to our divine source.

So manifestation is recognized for what it is—higher consciousness longing to experience itself. This very longing is the reason we are. It constitutes the root vibration of the universe. It is the prana that breathes life into things and the universal laws that establish the cyclical nature of existence. To embrace the wonder with which consciousness continually manifests and celebrate the perpetual state of flux that is the mark of this manifest world, whilst being rooted in pure consciousness, this is the freedom the yogi strives for.

HISTORICAL ROOTS

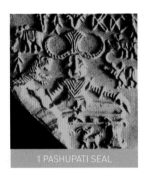

1 PASHUPATI SEAL

Yoga originated in ancient India and is the sum total of practices that seek to connect the soul with the divine ground of being. Although from a traditional perspective yoga is eternal and does not have a beginning point in time, historically it began when human beings set out to cultivate practices that would result in a direct encounter with the ultimate reality. Why do we exist? What happens at death? What is the true nature of reality, the individual spirit, and the cosmic supersoul? As these questions cannot be answered by mere speculation; some sort of practice had to be developed to enlighten the mind to ultimate truth. The system and lifestyle that was thus revealed as conducive to spiritual self-realization came to be referred to as yoga.

The earliest civilizations known to historians are those of ancient Egypt and the Nile, Mesopotamia, the Indus Valley, and China. Agriculture started before 5000 BCE in South Asia, and circa 3000 BCE villages spread down to the Indus Valley. The most famous of the early urban settlements are Harappa and Mohenjo Daro in what is now northwest India and Pakistan, which experienced their heyday from 2600 to 1900 BCE. These societies seemed to be very egalitarian, consisting of mostly traders and artisans. They established an extensive maritime trade network, with links to Afghanistan, the coastal regions of Persia, northern and central India, and Mesopotamia. The reasons behind the gradual decline of the

Indus-Saraswati civilization between 1800 and 1700 BCE are still a topic of debate, but climate change was probably the main deciding factor, with the disappearance of substantial portions of the Ghaggar-Hakra river system (which is identified with the Vedic Saraswati river). Seals depicting a figure standing on its head and one sitting cross-legged were found at Mohenjo Daro, indicating that some form of yoga asana was practiced here. A figure seated in *Siddhasana*, or even the advanced *Mulabandhasana* (SEE ILL.1), wearing elaborate horned headgear and surrounded by animals, is widely regarded as an early depiction of the god Shiva in his aspect as Pashupati, "lord of creatures". Inscriptions found on seals, ceramic pots, and other materials have led scholars to characterize the Indus Valley Civilization as a literate society. To date, however, these inscriptions have not been deciphered, and some scholars believe that these symbols did not encode language, but that they represent a variety of nonlinguistic sign systems used extensively in the Near East.

This remains an enigma to historians, as India holds the great cultural heritage of the Vedas, which were composed in Sanskrit. Up until the early 1980s, it was widely thought that the inhabitants of the Indus Valley were Dravidians, who were pushed out by marauding tribes that belonged to an Aryan race that spoke Indo-European languages and went on to establish the Vedic culture. This theory is now largely refuted, as there is no evidence of such migration, brutal invasion, or sudden appearance of racially different human remains. It is more likely that the northwestern Indians of the time simply migrated towards the nearby fertile Gangetic plains in search of greener pastures. Whether the Vedic culture was an import or native to the subcontinent is still open to debate, but a good case can be made for the latter theory. The Indus-Saraswati civilization displayed many crossovers with Vedic culture such as the presence of fire-altars, the symbol of a bull engraved on hundreds of seals, the cult of a mother-goddess, the Shiva-like deity, and of course the depiction of yogic postures as well as certain symbols used in later Indian culture, such as the *trishula* (three-spear or trident), the swastika, the pipal tree, or the endless knot design. They did however eat beef and bury their dead, which does not correspond with later Hindu practices. Even more baffling is that the Sanskrit language, with its linguistic affinity to European languages, is strangely absent. David Frawley argues that in the oldest Vedic Sanskrit we in fact find similar sounds to that of Dravidian languages that are alien to the Indo-European tongue. This would indicate that the two language groups in their origin emanated from a common root and that "the Aryans and Dravidians are part of the same culture and we need not speak of them as separate"[1].

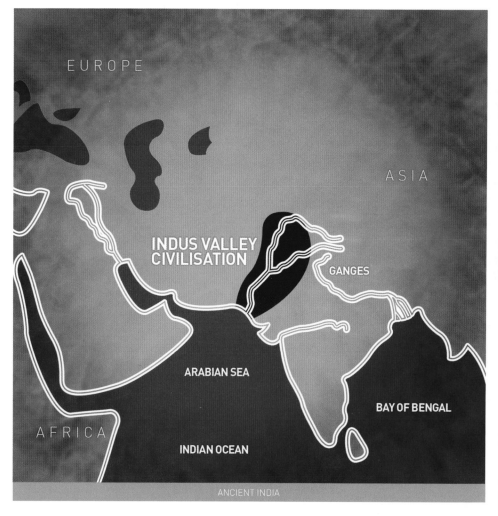
ANCIENT INDIA

IMPORTANT SCRIPTURES

The earliest form of the Vedic canon, the Rigveda, dates at least as far back as 1500 BCE. The Vedas are Sanskrit hymns, channeled directly by the rishis, or seers, and handed down as sacred and secret knowledge within the priestly fold, later to become the Brahmin caste. The Vedas contain mainly ritualistic formulas, chants, but also some pragmatic advice. Ritual was regarded as vital in sustaining the universal order. Many of the Gods referred to here are connected to the Greek-Roman pantheon, the result of an active cultural exchange along these important trade routes. The Brahmanas of circa 800 to 500 BCE, commentaries on the four Vedas, expanded the systemization of sacrificial ritual. These thus represent an early form of religious practice, the aim of which was to appease the gods, and moreover a political tool that retained the ability to do so in the hands of the priests who held this secret knowledge.

Parallel to this strand of thought, a genuinely mystical tradition developed that came to be integrated in yoga practice. As the Vedas were learned by heart through repeated recitation of the sacred teachings codified in mantras, it is here that the importance of sound becomes so pertinent. *Mantra* is derived from the Sanskrit word *manas*, or mind, and the suffix -*tra* may denote a "getting beyond", a "tool" and "instrument", or simply to "liberate". A mantra refers to a sacred word or words whose sound vibration takes the chanter beyond the limits of his or her conditioned mind. The power behind speech was regarded as an aspect of Brahma, the force or potentiality behind everything. Thus in about 1000 BCE, we see a new spiritual sentiment arise and a quest for oneness being expressed in the Upanishads (also referred to as Vedanta, or "end of the Vedas") and a definite move away from ritual towards philosophy. This eventually developed into the Hindu doctrine of Atman-Brahma, which holds that the human soul (*Atman*) is in essence one with ultimate reality (*Brahma*). By this time, the word *yoga* increasingly denotes a mental attitude toward things that leads to the realization of this oneness. In the later Maitri Upanishads, a sixfold path of yoga is outlined, which can be regarded as a precursor to Patanjali's "Eight Limbs".

In the epic scripture Mahabharata (eighth to sixth century BCE), which contains the famous and possibly older Bhagavad Gita, Samkhya and Yoga are mentioned as one philosophical school. Samkhya is one of the oldest systems of philosophy in India and the worldview it presents is implicit in classical yoga philosophy. Samkhya describes the condition and evolution of the universe, based on the fundamental duality of purusha (spirit), and prakriti, (matter). Purusha is the knower, on which the manifestation of the material universe, prakriti, relies. Prakriti is divided into twenty-four categories or "evolutes", each of them consisting of varying distributions of the three "strands", or gunas: sattva, rajas, and tamas.

Tamas is the force of consumption; it is heavy, dark, and causes inertia. Rajas is responsible for activity, expends energy, and is therefore cause for passion, heat, and motion. Sattva is the illuminating quality of all things, radiant, pure, and enlightening. The gunas always exist together and their interaction makes for the constant state of evolution of the universe. Without purusha however, the gunas would be in a state of balance and the universe would be unmanifest. This potential condition is referred to as *mula prakriti*, or primal nature. Fundamental to the Samkhya worldview is the idea of *satkaryavada*, which means that effects are implicit in causes. The universe has no beginning or end, every period of evolution being followed by a period of dissolution in a continuous cycle. Purusha, being pure spirit, is not subject to change, and it is only by purusha that prakriti is infused with consciousness and thus evolves from its potential, latent form to manifest being. Yoga embraces the metaphysics of the Samkhya philosophy, but adds God (Ishvara) and purusha to prakriti's twenty-four evolutes.

Building on Samkhya philosophy in his Yoga Sutras, Patanjali indicates the method and means of liberation—freedom from the deluded identification with prakriti towards a realization of purusha as the true self. The Yoga Sutras were probably compiled around the third century CE in the Gupta period, although many historians set a much earlier date around the second century BCE. There is also much confusion as to who Patanjali was, as many other important scriptures, including one of Sanskrit grammar and another on Ayurveda have been attributed to this prolific sage-scholar. In sculpture, Patanjali is depicted as half-snake, half-man (or naga), as he came to be regarded in Indian mythology as an incarnation of the thousand-headed naga Ananta, (meaning "endless"), who serves as Vishnu's serpent-couch, guarding the world's treasures.

The Yoga Sutras are divided into four *padas*, or chapters, the fourth often regarded as a later addition. Patanjali's comprehensive system is referred to as Raja Yoga, or the "royal path". Many commentaries were written to reveal the meaning of these terse verses, the most acclaimed one being Vyasa from the fifth or sixth century CE.

Samadhi Pada, the first chapter, focuses on liberation and investigates the vrttis, or inner fluctuations, that disturb the mind, and how these get in the way of self-realization. Patanjali posits an absolute true consciousness, *Ishvara* (or God), and outlines the way to merge with the Supreme.

Sadhana Pada, the second chapter, addresses practice and outlines the all-important Eight Limbs of Yoga, Ashtanga Yoga, which to this day form the basis for a yogi's way of life and practice. The first four limbs are referred to as the outer limbs, while the other four represent the inner limbs. In other words, we are first taught how to deal with the world around us and maintain the physical and energetic body. After this we are shown how to control the senses, emotions, and thoughts.

The first two limbs outline a lifestyle conducive to spiritual advancement.

Yama means "restraint" or "abstention", of which there are five types:
Ahimsa: nonviolence
Satya: truthfulness
Asteya: not stealing
Brahmacharya: continence or abstention from sexual misconduct
Aparigraha: renouncing possessions

Niyama means "observance". There are also five types:.
Shaucha: purity
Santosha: contentment
Tapas: austerities
Svadyaya: study of the self
Ishvara Pranidhana: dedication to God, or that which you regard as divine.

The third and fourth limbs advise the spiritual seeker to make the body strong and to maximize its energetic capacity.

Asana literally means "seat" and is most often translated as "posture". *Sthira sukham asanam* (Posture should be steady and pleasant). This is the only direct reference Patanjali makes to the physical practice of yoga, and some scholars such as Georg Feuerstein even believe the entire Ashtanga section was interpolated into the Sutras. Nevertheless, this brief statement does encapsulate the essence of asana practice, and moreover indicates a complete way of life. "Posture should be steady and pleasant", can be viewed simply as a guideline for how the yogi should sit for meditation, or a description of the qualities that should be cultivated in the body in any posture. Yet, it also indicates the attitude a yogi will take towards life and relationships in general, one of total mindfulness without loss of inner joy. Whether it pertains to others or oneself, full effort should be made to live by one's truth, while sustaining a level of comfort that ensures continuity.

Pranayama means both "restraint" and "harnessing" of vital life force, or prana. This is done through specific exercises in breath-control. The acknowledgement of the breath as not only a reservoir of life force, but as a practical link between the mind and a state of pure consciousness beyond thought, is of great significance, as it preempts later traditions that make breathing exercises their key feature. (See Chapter 5)

The fifth and sixth limbs explain how to turn and hold the attention inward.

Pratyahara denotes a control of the senses, pulling them away like a turtle pulls in its head and limbs. In other words, our preoccupation with outer stimuli is held in check and we free ourselves from distraction.

Dharana means "concentration," which is the result of fixing one's attention on a single object, which can be either external or internal. Thus we control the activities of the "monkey-mind" by offering it a single branch to cling to, resulting in one-pointed focus, ekagrata.

The final two limbs pertain to the deeper states that can be achieved through regular meditation practice.

Dhyana, or meditation, results from a state of total absorption in the object of focus. Here there is no self-awareness and the duality between perceiver and the perceived is overcome.

Samadhi, or enlightenment, finally occurs when, through the nondual state of absorption, a transcendental shift in consciousness results. It cannot be captured in words, as these can only describe conceptual reality, but bliss, ultimate deliverance from the illusion of separation, and thus freedom from suffering indicate some of the aspects of this superconscious state.

Vibhuti Pada, the third chapter of the Yoga Sutras, can be translated as the chapter on the "powers of manifestation." As vibhuti refers to the ashes from a yogi's sacred fire, it denotes the indestructible essence of things. Here the siddhis (supernatural powers) that a yogi can attain are revealed. These are a result of the prolonged ability to hold all three of the last limbs (dharana, dhyana, and samadhi) simultaneously, which is referred to as samyama.

Kaivalya Pada, the fourth chapter, describes the liberated state of moksha, when the mind is free from karmic impressions as a result of yoga and meditation practice. *Kaivalya* literally means "isolated" or "detached" and refers to the emancipation of consciousness from the fluctuating mind-states that are a result of causes and conditions. In the independent state of absolute true consciousness, the mind dwells in its own pure nature and the gunas return to their source.

In its systemization, Patanjali's Eight Limbs of Yoga echo the Buddhist Noble Eightfold Path, and many of its concepts show Buddhist influence. In turn, the Yoga Sutras offered a consistent philosophical basis for yoga practice and paved the way for the later Hindu and Buddhist Tantra (Vajrayana) yoga schools.

One of the most important and early systems of Hindu philosophy is Vedanta, which its most famous interpreter, Shankaracharya, developed into Advaita Vedanta in the eighth century. Yoga philosophy is regarded as *dvaita* (dual), in that through sadhana, spiritual practice, and the illumination it brings, a transformation in our essential state of being takes place, which leads to enlightenment. This implies a process, which the *advaita* (nondual) traditions do without. Brahma is regarded as the sole reality, and this ultimate reality is impersonal, nameless, and formless. Shankaracharya explained that we are already part of this reality, but due to a temporary state of illusion (maya), which serves as a sort of superimposition (*adyasa*), we are blinded. The way to freedom (moksha) is through knowledge. Advaita Vedanta as an Indian philosophy came to be widely recognized in the West, when Vivekananda spoke to the Parliament of World Religions in America in 1896.

Current-day Hinduism has no single founder and refers to a very wide variety of beliefs and practices, the outlining of which would be beyond the scope of this book. Although it famously displays a whole pantheon of gods, in its essence it is monotheistic, in that these gods are regarded as emanations of the one undifferentiated and eternal essence, or supersoul, Brahman. Brahman manifests in many personalized forms to allow human beings, who rely on limited faculties of perception, to connect to the divine. Bhakti, the devotional strand of yoga, and regular practice of puja, worship of one's chosen deity, is central to Hindu life. Hinduism today can be broadly divided into three main sects, who respectively worship Shiva ("the destroyer," the divine in its fierce aspect responsible for transcendental wisdom and yoga), Vishnu ("the sustainer," who keeps the cosmic order of the universe by manifesting in various forms on earth), or Shakti (the feminine principle often associated with the generative force of nature). Traditionally, Brahma took the place of "the creator" and together with Vishnu and Shiva, represented the endless cycle of time.

The schools of thought that culminated in Patanjali's compilation of the Yoga Sutras belong to India's orthodox tradition of religio-philosophy. Hinduism embraces the ideas set forth in the scriptures mentioned above, but differentiates between the Vedas and Upanishads that are regarded as *shruti* (heard), implying a direct transmission of eternal truths, and those that are *smriti*, (remembered), derived from man's insight and experience, the most notable of these being the epics Mahabharata and Ramayana.

The story of the Bhagavad Gita, the "Song of the Lord" as recorded in the Mahabharata, is said to contain the essence of the Vedas. The Gita is a story about Arjuna, a kshatriya, or warrior prince. Pitched for one of the greatest battles in the history of ancient India, he is plagued by sudden pangs of doubt, and laying down his weapons, refuses to fight. His charioteer turns out to be no less than Krishna, an avatar, or incarnation, of Vishnu. In his discourse, Krishna offers to reveal the quintessential secrets of yoga. He urges Arjuna to fight, as this is in accordance with his dharma, (duty or truth). He further explains that actions are free from karmic (retributive) charge if they are carried out without desire for the fruits of the act, but instead in an attitude of dedication to "the Lord" or Ishvara, the Supreme Being. This definition of yoga marked by karma (action) and bhakti (devotion) exposes a trend towards integrating spiritual aims into the worldly domain of a society that upheld an increasingly strict caste system.

It is important to understand that there existed a parallel stream of spirituality that consisted of an ascetic lifestyle and a renouncing of society. It is here that most of the physical practices of yoga known to us today have their roots. The phenomenon of asceticism can be found in all cultures, but the tradition of renunciation was particularly strong in India and is still practiced there today. Terms used for ascetics are *saddhu*, *sannyasin*, *sramana*, and *yogi*. The word sramana is derived from the Sanskrit *shram*, (to exert effort or perform austerity) and is linguistically related to the word *shaman*. Sramana sects are known to have been active as early as the fifth century BCE, representing an egalitarian mystical counterculture to that of Vedic ritual performed solely by the Brahmin priestly elite. A person becomes a saddhu when in a specific ritual of renunciation under a chosen guru, or spiritual teacher, he or she abandons all forms of identity. In the fourth century BCE, the grammarian Panini refers in his "Ashtadhyayi" (meaning "Eight Chapters") to codes of conduct for such mendicants, and Patanjali the grammarian in the second century BCE mentions in his "Great Commentary" (Mahabhashya) *Shivabhagavatas*, who he describes as wandering ascetics wearing animal skins and carrying iron lances. These were most probably Shaiva ascetics (worshippers of Shiva), or Pashupatas, who were renowned for their antisocial behavior and took their name from Shiva's epithet as "Lord of the Beasts." The aim of moksha, or liberation, was regarded as difficult to attain within the framework of normal worldly existence. The penance these saddhus received from their crude living conditions was said to help them attain supernatural powers, or *siddhis*, such as being able to mind-read, become invisible, or walk on water. By the grace of Shiva, they would eventually merge with Him.

By the thirteenth or fourteenth century CE, the Naths (literally, "lords"), another Shaiva sect renowned for their heterodox behavior and warrior background, began to propagate Hatha Yoga practice in various scriptures. The most famous of these is the Hatha Yoga Pradipika ("Light on Hatha Yoga"), consisting of slokas, or verses, that are attributed to the sage Gorakshanath. *Hatha* means "force" or "exertion," and in India refers to the most rigorous yoga path. Texts with a particularly New Age slant state that ha- refers to the sun, the male, or *yang* aspect, and -*tha* to the moon, the female, or *yin* aspect, which would mean that the two together balance two opposite energies. The perfection of the human body was thought to have such a transformational effect on a person's state of consciousness that it could make them a jivanmukta, or one who is "liberated in life."

The Nath tradition assimilated practices drawn from alchemy, Tantra, yoga, and Ayurveda. Although not entirely coherent, in the Hatha Yoga Pradipika we find a complete system of cleansing the body through six actions called the *Shat Karma Kriyas*. (See Chapter 5) These make reference to the most key elements of human subtle anatomy, as well as to descriptions of *pranayama*, breathing exercises in conjunction with *bandhas* (locks) and mudras (seals). Again the expressed aim was the acquisition of *siddhis*, or supernatural powers, samadhi being regarded as not just a state of blissful deliverance, but also the source of these powers that would lead to an increase in *bhoga*, or enjoyment of life.

MAJOR CURRENT STREAMS OF HATHA YOGA

Nowadays anybody who decides to take up yoga practice will face an almost confusing variety of options. Below, I briefly outline the main streams active today and attempt to place them into one of the main lineages. Keep in mind that this is an oversimplification and you would do well to research the relevant schools for more information before you make your choice. It is hoped that by using the Quantum Method you will ultimately be able to identify what is useful from these varying styles, and thus select what to integrate into your own personal practice. Again let me make clear here that in the context of this book I have chosen to primarily list yoga traditions that have asana-*pranayama* practice as one of their central features. It is important to bear in mind that in other yoga traditions, bhakti (devotion), karma (charitable acts), jnana (study of the ancient scriptures), and nada (the use of sound) constitute the essence of their particular paths.

Possibly the most important figure to have had a huge impact on yoga as it is practiced internationally today was Shri Tirumalai Krishnamacharya (1891–1989). He managed to harmoniously combine an understanding of asana practice, which during his time was affected by the influence of British physical and military education, with a deep understanding of the more esoteric aspects of yoga then current in Tibet. He did much of his research by observing these forgotten practices preserved only in remote areas of the Himalayas, without losing sight of the orthodoxy of Patanjali's teachings. His four main students all went on to form influential schools of their own.

B. K. S. Iyengar teaches his Iyengar style in Pune, India and internationally, with a focus on precise structure, alignment, and the extensive use of props to allow any kind of body to gain the benefits of yoga practice. Patthabi Jois, active both in Mysore, India and internationally, has experienced great success with the Ashtanga Vinyasa Yoga system, a challenging dynamic form that contains four main sequences (sometimes also split into six sequences). Ashtanga encourages physical adjustments and its key elements are *ujaii* (victorious) breathing, *bandhas* (locks), *vinyasa* (breath-synchronized movement), and *drishti* (fixed eye gaze). T. K. V. Desikachar, Krishnamacharya's son, resides in Chennai, from where his teachings have spread internationally. His is a slower approach that is best taught one-on-one, as the cultivation of correct breathing through movement forms its key element. The enigmatic Indra Devi was Krishnamacharya's first Western pupil and went on to teach many famous students in her studio in Hollywood. In later life she moved to Argentina where she formed the Indra Devi Foundation, which is still active after she passed away in 2002. "Movements in yoga," she explained, "are harmonious, slow, soft, plastic, relaxed, always conscious, and require a permanent and active mental participation. The whole work rests on the dialectic tension-relaxation."[2] Many new styles of yoga have evolved from Krishnamacharya's heritage, with the aim of making these teachings more accessible to contemporary understanding. Such modern schools include Anusara, Yin, and Jivamukti, the latter having also been inspired by the more devotional Shivananda approach.

The Shivananda tradition has been extremely influential, with its freer style of asana practice that focuses on *Suryanamaskara* (Sun Salutations) and twelve basic postures. It encourages intermittent relaxation between postures. Shivananda's approach, with its emphasis on *kriyas*, mudras, *pranayama*, and visualization meditation, is more holistic than the previous asana-focused schools. Swami Satchidananda integrated Shivananda with the Integral Yoga tradition that had been pioneered by Sri Aurobindo Gosh. Swami Satyananda Saraswati was a disciple of Shivananda and started the Bihar School of Yoga, a veritable yoga university from which a prolific array of yoga books has facilitated many students' understanding. Swami Brahmananda Saraswati developed the transcendental meditation methods and today Deepak Chopra is one of the more prominent figures to have studied in this lineage. Kripalu Yoga, mostly active in the United States, is yet another school that grew out of the Hindu spiritual renaissance and the revival of Hatha Yoga that began in the 1950s and brought these varied traditions to the West. One of the more recently successful offshoots from this lineage is Bikram Yoga, which has a set sequence of asana and is done in artificially heated rooms.

Kundalini Yoga, which sees its roots in the Sikh tradition, includes a lot of advanced *pranamyama* and mantra recitation. Introduced to the West by Yogi Bhajan in 1969, Kundalini Yoga promises to accelerate the transformative process of yoga practice through techniques that stimulate the spine and endocrine system to awaken this dormant reservoir of prana within (see Chapter 3) and lead to psycho-spiritual growth. The Tibetan tradition of yoga is interesting in that its isolated geographic location, prior to the Chinese invasion in 1950, ensured that its treasure of ancient spiritual wisdom, much of which had its roots in mainland India, remained intact and untouched by foreign influence. Kriya Yoga is today possibly best known for its famous adherent Paramhansa Yogananda, who wrote the popular *Autobiography of a Yogi*.

Whatever style, tradition, or teachings you explore, bear in mind that the fundamental truth that forms the basis of all spiritual quests is very clear and simple. It is the insight that everything you need to know you can find within. Yoga can give you the tools to uncover this treasure, and a good teacher will inspire you by their own efforts and show you how to use them, but only you really know where to start digging.

YOGA AND QUANTUM PHYSICS

THE TRUE NATURE OF REALITY

"QUANTUM PHYSICS, VERY SUCCINCTLY SPEAKING, IS THE PHYSICS OF POSSIBILITIES."[3]

Although I am far from being a quantum physicist, I do want to make a few remarks about the correlation I perceive with yoga. A basic premise of quantum physics is that consciousness seems to manifest our reality. This insight echoes not only the teachings of early Indian thinkers who informed the worldview set forth by the Samkhya philosophy and later adopted in Patanjali's Yoga Sutras, but it also reflects the experience of any yogi following a sustained practice. In the Samkhya cosmology, once the process of manifestation has begun, the ability to sense matter evolves before matter itself does. So, for example, the sense of smell evolves before odor. Our ability to perceive a thing develops before the thing itself comes into existence.

Einstein coined the term *superimposition* to describe the fact that on a subatomic level, the building blocks of our material universe can exist both as particles and waveforms at the same time. Electrons are not bound by space-time restrictions, as they can be everywhere in the universe simultaneously. However, as soon as one attempts to measure this phenomenon, the particle leaves this quantum dimension and collapses into a single aspect of space-time

reality. In other words, a particle that previously existed in a state of infinite quantum potentiality, through the interference of observation, materializes in just one of the infinite possibilities. The yogis' ability to merge with the quantum field of infinite possibilities results in their attainment of *siddhis*, or supernatural powers. How do they bypass the interference of observation that causes particles to lose their capacity to superimpose and manifest as fixed matter limited by time and space?

Quantum physics has scientifically proven what the yogis, Buddhas, and mystics have always taught, namely that the reality we perceive as being "out there," in a fixed state, is in fact an illusion. Instead, what we are actually dealing with is a field of infinite possibilities, which is in a constant state of flux. The reality we perceive is what our brain has come to assume is there. Our experience therefore is merely a result of conditioning.

What interests us here though is what determines how we experience this reality. "Our minds are also quantum-measuring devices," writes Stephen Linsteadt. "Our thoughts create electromagnetic waves that have the ability to induce electrical impulses in neurons. . . . Our cells respond and entrain to our CEM-field by adjusting their quantum-measuring apparatuses to select that which conforms to our conscious or sub-conscious expectations."[4] Linsteadt goes on to attribute disease to a cell's "distorted quantum perspective."

Yogi mystics posit against this illusory conditioning a direct experience of reality as a nondual state of consciousness. This *bypassing* of the mind, which results from systematic techniques to stop the mind's inner turbulence by temporarily suspending thought, is the only way we can catch a glimpse of how things really are. This begs the question, who and what then is experiencing this ultimate reality? If we have always attributed the faculty of observation to the mind, and if the ultimate observer is not to be found here, where is it then? In the domain of Indian mysticism, this witness, or *sakshi*, was likened to Lord Shiva sitting on the top of Mount Kailash, unaffected by the harsh conditions, self-sufficient, totally still, and simply observing. The answer quantum physics will give you, however, is simple: we do not know. No matter how sophisticated the scientific instruments and how deeply we have penetrated the human brain and the rest of the body, there is no ultimate observer to be found. As Erwin Shroedinger insists: "Science cannot touch it."[5] In a sense therefore, the greatest contribution that quantum physics has made is that we now definitely know what we do not know. There are limits to what the mind alone can access, and science can, by definition, only ever be a product of the mind. It has not proven the insights of the mystics, but it has handed questions pertaining to the Ultimate, based on the epistemological limitations of science, firmly over to them.

THE QUANTUM METHOD OF YOGA

The way in which we experience the world changes as we refine our approach to it. Any type of asana-*pranayama* will do this to a degree, but if you turn your practice into a conscious act of self-healing that involves an active dialogue between body/energy and mind/heart, the results will be more powerful. In the context of yoga, as well as quantum physics, the body (or matter in general) cannot be spoken of as divorced from energy. Though asana practice results in tangible results similar to those of conventional exercise routines, the energetic realignment that it brings is empirically undeniable and scientifically measurable, especially when coupled with *pranayama*.

Quantum physics has revealed that matter consists of spaces held together by energy. The thing that is more "real," in the sense that it informs the qualities and characteristics of a thing, is this energy, not the object itself. That energy responds immediately when it comes into contact with other force fields, and our mind, though not itself the source, directs energy. Hence, as soon as the instruments of perception are directed to a thing, that thing responds and changes;

so it is with the body in yoga. This is why for our practice to be truly effective and transformative, it has to make room for such interactivity. Furthermore, once we imbue our sadhana with greater consciousness, we will become skilled at sustaining this same level of awareness in all our actions. The importance of intention takes on a whole new dimension, and this realization will cause fundamental change and improvement in our lives and that of others.
We hereby truly take responsibility for our health and happiness. Even if we always intellectually understood the karmic laws of cause and effect, it is only when we begin to actually observe the connections that we attain some measure of control over our destiny. Quantum Yoga provides us with the tools that allow us to move in this direction. The first step is simple. Learn to listen and pay attention to what is really going on.

THE POWER OF MANIFESTATION

In recent years, films such as *What the Bleep!?* and *The Secret* and bestselling books like *Ask and it is Given* have opened the insights of quantum physics to a wider audience (even though some critics discarded much of the quantum insights presented in these movies as misinformed). In itself this is a great achievement and will hopefully inspire more people to undertake further study of the subject. The danger of a superficial propagation of the subject however is that the

basic focus seems to always remain, how can we manifest our deepest desires? And the desires often proposed here are based on an unashamed consumer mentality, such as how to get that new sports car you always wanted or that condo in Miami.

Implicit in this modern approach is the feeling that we do not already have all we need and must thus acquire the skill to manifest what we want by using the laws of attraction. Indeed, this capacity is nothing other than those supernatural powers or *siddhis* the ancient scriptures promise. But with that promise comes a warning: such powers can cement the control of the ego and create strong attachments that will represent a hindrance to the final liberated state, free from desire. The problem may not be that we cannot get what we want, but that we always linger in a state of wanting. So what if you get that new sports car, won't you then want more? The circumstances of our lives determine its quality only to a limited degree, as satisfaction from achievement is more often than not short-lived and usually gets replaced by another desire.

A key spiritual insight communicated by the yogi mystics is that perfection is in the now. Desire, per se, represents a projection into the future and a reinforcing of the ego-mind. This does posit a causal contradiction in that the initial motivation that leads to spiritual practice is in itself a desire to be enlightened. A solution can be found perhaps if we learn to differentiate between a desire for sense satisfaction and outer recognition, as opposed to a longing to realize the true nature of being without being motivated by secondary effects that pertain to worldly success. Once we attain cosmic consciousness, we realize that enlightenment represents the ability to truly inhabit the moment. Ultimately, yoga is that state where you need nothing.

Nevertheless, as nature expresses herself through constant change and we are part of her, yearning and ambition have their place. Yet, as yogis, it is of utmost importance to identify what our true aspirations are. The psychic capacity that Quantum Yoga equips the practitioner with really does enable one to transform one's life. Therefore, be careful what you wish for! Are those desires really yours or are they a result of ambitions you have been conditioned to have? Will the fulfillment of those desires really raise the quality of your life? In this so-called communication age, what the media is constantly communicating to us via its various channels is more often than not rooted in lack, and exploits our natural fear for survival. Therefore, becoming clear about what it is one really needs and truly wants is an essential prerequisite. Otherwise you may receive these precious teachings and gain the power to manifest, but end up with something that does not feed your soul.

The teaching of the gunas can be very useful in identifying those things we should set about manifesting into our lives as spiritual seekers. Remember that the gunas, the basic qualities that make up prakriti (matter, that is, everything that is not spirit) always coexist, but in varying distributions. Sattva is the enlightening quality in all things—that which brings knowledge, clarity, and health. Everything has a sattvic side to it. As yogis, we recognize and cultivate the sattva in things. Quantum physics in turn dictates that like will attract like. No matter what your circumstances are at present, if you focus on and feel gratitude for the things that you have, which are good in your life—and "good" in the context of yoga means that which supports your spiritual aspirations—more of it will come your way. This can of course mean that if there are lessons to be learned, they will come around hard and fast. I have heard many serious yogis lament that they just can't get away with anything since they stepped on the path. Indeed your karma will speed up with the growing awareness that yoga brings. Why is that?

Karma literally means "action." Actions are threefold: physical, mental, and somnial. All these will produce forces of retribution. The more consciousness you bring into your actions, the greater their force will be. The laws of cause and effect are inevitable and if you live more mindfully, you will soon recognize the connections. Getting away from victimization and taking responsibility for one's life is a logical result of this heightened level of awareness, and the power this process eventually grants is remarkable. If you have a regular sadhana to fall back on and moreover have been lucky enough to have found a guru you can trust, then you will be able to bravely face the karmic repercussions of past deeds and get on with cultivating a life that leads to freedom.

"Relax, Nothing is under Control!"[6]

Life is full of mystery. Even when we think that we have gained some clarity, that we are more in control, an unpredictable turn in events will change everything. Being free doesn't mean having the complete handle on reality. No, it is more likely to mean that we resonate with its profound mystery, that we rejoice in its many surprises, and that we humbly go about our lives accepting that these things have been manifested by ourselves, even if those karmic seeds were sown eons ago.

THE PRACTICAL RELEVANCE OF ENERGY AND MATTER

Under *The Quantum Science of Spirituality* (p.62), I have given an autobiographical account of how asana-*pranayama* practice served as the first direct indication that the insights of quantum physics—namely that energy becomes more tangible than matter itself—could be experienced firsthand in the body. This has certainly been the case in my body, where

the avalanche of energetic stirring has sometimes been frighteningly explosive. Luckily I have had the knowledge of the scriptures, the support of nature, and the loving guidance of my gurus to fall back on.

Sometimes when I adjust my students, they later ask me how I knew that a particular body part was in need of attention. I always have to confess that it is not a result of a scientific understanding of anatomy and physiology, nor had my attention been with their every movement throughout the class. It is more that I intuitively perceive the areas where the energy is blocked, and my hands are drawn to them. Quantum theory speaks of virtual particles that cannot be measured, but we know they are there, as we can observe their effects on the measurable mass. In yoga too we work with variables that are not always directly perceivable, but can be intuited. We do see the obvious benefits to the physical body, the emotions, and the state of mind of yoga students.

If we let go of the antiquated understanding of matter, which viewed the atom as the ultimate substantial entity, and embrace what modern science has come to reveal, we soon realize that this world of fixed objects that we have come to accept as real is not such. Even the nucleus of the atom has no ultimate substance; in fact matter is held together purely by energetic forces attracting or repelling each other. Matter is, as it were, hollow and totally subject to the energy that holds it together. When we begin to work with the body-mind complex in such a conscious and systematic manner as we do in Quantum Yoga, and we furthermore embrace that we are working with prana, which is the essence of life that connects us all, then it comes as little surprise that the resulting experiences take us beyond this limited perception of matter as a fixed substance, towards a true and immediate realization of the nature of reality, which is one of an interactive energetic field imbued with consciousness. In the search for the ultimate observer we realize that God is not outside of us, or even somewhere hidden within us, but that the very yearning to know God is God.

"When he thus yokes himself continuously, the yogin of restrained thought attains to the peace that lies in me, beyond nirvana," Lord Krishna promises Arjuna in the Bhagavad Gita.

WHAT WE NOW KNOW IS THAT WE DON'T KNOW

The main contribution of quantum physics has been to prove that there are things we simply cannot grasp with the logical mind. There are limits to the level of conceptual understanding we can access. This is for the pure reason that the mind is directly involved in the manifestation of reality, so there is no way to divide the two. How can the mind know what the mind perceives, when in the very act of perceiving, it is shaping the reality it believes to be perceiving? The further we

explore the workings of the universe through scientific means, the more we become aware of the fact that there are limits to our capacity to understand the true nature of reality, as the very act of perception is part of its creation. Yogic insight is the result of direct nondual perception or pure consciousness that is only accessible when the mind has been brought to a state of complete stillness, and therefore its epistemology goes beyond anything that science and measurable truth can access. Science is about measurement. It can, for instance, measure the effects that advanced states of consciousness have on the various cortexes of a seasoned meditator's brain. Through experiments and the study of statistics, we can even deduce that a large amount of people practicing these techniques for stilling the mind have a direct effect on their immediate environment. However, science cannot describe, prove, replicate, or quantify what the actual experience is in a state of samadhi, nor can it really attribute the experience to any particular faculty. The big difference between the classic deterministic view of the world and the new dimension of quantum physics is that we now recognize, based on the facts we have gathered and studied with our logical minds, that there are limitations to what we can mentally capture and explain. Absolute understanding lies beyond the conceptual reality we create in our minds.

In his book *Quantum Questions*, Ken Wilber explores the links between quantum physics and spirituality when he warns his readers not to confuse modern scientific findings with the insights of the mystics, as this one-size-fits-all New Age approach could actually backfire and undermine spiritual truth. "There is the great difference between the old and new physics," he writes. "Both are dealing with shadows, but the old physics didn't recognize that fact."[7]

When one studies their writings, it is remarkable how most of the great quantum physicists seem to unanimously return to the same conclusion. Namely that to grasp the very essence of reality goes beyond the realm of science, and can only be realized through direct experience as the result of spiritual practice. In Eddington's words:

"Briefly the position is this. We have learnt that the exploration of the external world by the methods of physical science leads not to a concrete reality but to a shadow world of symbols, beneath which those methods are unadapted for penetrating . . . Feeling that there must be more behind, we return to our starting point in human consciousness—the one centre where more might become known. There [in immediate inward consciousness] we find other stirrings, other revelations (true or false) than those conditioned by the world of symbols . . . Physics most strongly insists that its methods do not penetrate behind the symbolism. Surely then that mental and spiritual nature of ourselves, known in our minds by an intimate contact transcending the methods of physics, supplies just that . . . which science is admittedly unable to give."[8]

YET WE ALWAYS KNEW . . .

Yoga is about realizing the very grounds of reality, which are immeasurable and ineffable, because if the knower and the known become one, there can be no process of acquiring knowledge, but simply a state of knowing. Furthermore, if that "knowing" is a result of transcending all fluctuating mental states, then through the mastery of the yogic techniques realizing it may have been a result of many years of disciplined practice, the wisdom that is thus made conscious must be something that has always been there.

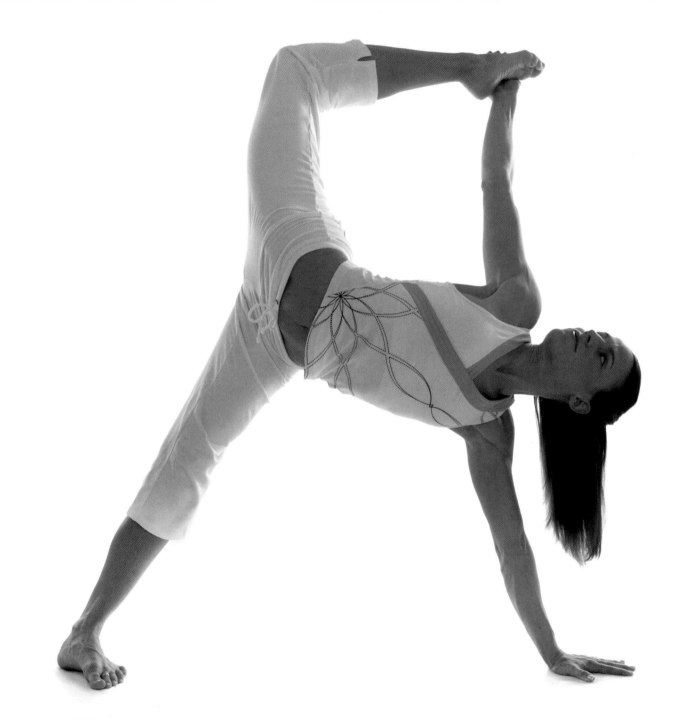

CHAPTER TWO
YOGA ANATOMY AND AYURVEDA

THE RELATIONSHIP BETWEEN GROSS AND SUBTLE ANATOMY

STHIRA SUKHAM ASANAM. "POSTURE SHOULD BE STEADY AND PLEASANT." (PATANJALI'S YOGA SUTRAS, II. 46)

A sana means "seat," "posture," "attitude," or "relationship." It is the third limb of Patanjali's eight-limbed system (Ashtanga). Correct asana practice increases strength, flexibility, fitness, vitality, joy (as it increases serotonin levels), and thus health in general. It leads to longevity and ensures a better quality of life. From the point of view of conventional exercise, Quantum Yoga offers all the usual benefits. It hardens the bones, strengthens muscles, stretches, and tones, increasing our range of movement and leaving the practitioner feeling and looking radiant and firm. As it works into the deeper layers of the muscles, it facilitates ideal posture and massages the organs, ensuring their efficient functioning. It heightens the capacity of the body to assimilate nutrients from food and expel what it no longer needs, thus increasing the metabolic rate. Quantum Yoga stimulates movement of blood and lymph and supports the biochemical balance ensured by functioning glands and regulated hormones. It stimulates and balances the sympathetic and parasympathetic nervous system as well. Many of these positive effects for the body are achieved through inversions, application of *bandhas*, or locks, stimulation of pressure points, and of course the control of the breath. On a physical level *pranayama* improves lung capacity, increases the oxygen supply to the blood and thereby all cells, exercises the diaphragm and thereby tones and massages the internal organs, allows for a greater release of toxins through the exhalation, and regulates the heartbeat.

There is a great debate in the world of fitness as to whether yoga answers the cardiovascular demands that ensure a healthy heart. The approach here is completely different, and dare I say more sophisticated, to that of conventional exercise, where the heart rate is deliberately brought up, leading to rapid breathing, profuse sweating, and increased pulse. Dynamic flowing forms of yoga without breath regulation and the application of *bandhas* does just that, but runs contrary to the higher aim of yoga. Its advantage over conventional exercise philosophy is revealed here. Quantum Yoga results in the usual physical responses of conventional exercise, but also provides the tools to slow down, and deepen and control the breath. This in turn will regulate the heart rate and keep the pulse down. In short, we are moving the body into unusual postures that require concentration, skill, and strength, but challenge it to remain calm and still. Once this skill is achieved in relation to our own body, mastery of any stressful situation becomes tangible.

One of the United Kingdom's leading personal trainers once caused an outcry in the yoga world by publishing an article that bore the heading, "Yoga does not make you fit." Anybody who has practiced Quantum or any other form of dynamic vinyasa yoga knows that it does make you fit, and far more deeply and lastingly than working out in a gym. More importantly, the above statement is missing the point altogether. Yoga's aim is not fitness. Practitioners who think so are shortchanging themselves. Yoga leads to union with the Absolute. Asana, *pranayama*, and *kriya* were not merely designed to strengthen the body, but to activate psychic powers. Furthermore, the physical and energetic alignment that consistent practice brings makes the body into a perfect vessel through which to experience exalted mind-states in meditation.

Another interesting anecdote happened at The Place, one of London's top dance schools, where I used to teach weekly yoga classes. The manager, a former professional ballet dancer, once revealed to me that he found yoga "just too hard." Coming from him, I found this very surprising. Surely ballet training must be really tough! Eventually I understood that especially for someone who comes from a performance background, yoga must seem utterly counterintuitive. You are trying to get into all these contorted shapes, but then you are told that the real challenge is to be able to relax in them!

From a biological perspective, human beings are ruled by the fight-or-flight reflex and equipped with a mind that is programmed for problem-solving. With regards to the preservation of humans as a species, especially in a cave-dwelling hunter-gatherer situation, the mental state and behavioral patterns predetermined by this biological conditioning are totally appropriate. Now, however, most of us are no longer concerned with mere survival on a daily basis. The practice of yoga indicates a way to exist beyond this conditioning. It comes as no surprise therefore that yoga made its first appearance in the early settlements of Harappa and Mohenjo Daro, when the introduction of agriculture allowed for a less primal lifestyle.

In the Yoga Sutras, Patanjali makes only one reference to asana, and it is widely accepted by academics that what he is referring to is the literal meaning of asana as "seat"—in this case how the yogi should sit for meditation. Nevertheless, if we apply his description to the physical body in general, the translation indicates that "posture should be steady and pleasant." In asana practice, we put the body into deliberately challenging positions, and yet aim to cultivate an attitude that is constantly dedicated and joyful. We apply ourselves completely and yet sustain a state of relative relaxation. Asana practice should thus never be aggressive or forceful, as this would be contrary to the principle of nonviolence (ahimsa) that is a prerequisite for a life of yoga. At the same time the attention should never be dissipated, as the greatest challenge of a spiritual life is that of total mindfulness. Ultimately in asana practice, the body becomes a training ground for sustaining such a relationship with all beings and things, one that is "skillfully nonchalant and yet ceaselessly concerned" (Prajnaparamita Sutra).

The breath is the key in monitoring this fine balance in our yoga practice. In dynamic asana, we apply *ujaii* breath and synchronize the controlled inner movement of the diaphragm with the outer physical movement of the body (*vinyasa*). *Ujaii pranayama* results in a constant smooth rasping sound, generated from a gentle contraction at the back of the throat, which should accompany you throughout any *vinyasa* practice. This soothing sound should translate the fine balance of *sthira* and *sukha*, as well as support concentration. In other words, the breath is strong and soft at the same time, and inhalation and exhalation of similar length and even intensity throughout (unless one has chosen to weave other specific *pranayamas* into the asana practice).

Psychologically what this means is that faced with any stressful situation, we can overcome our natural fight-or-flight reflex. Every time, whether we are stuck in a traffic jam or being shouted at by the boss, the system is releasing massive amounts of adrenaline. Unless used up physically, the adrenaline becomes stagnant and taxes the system. Through asana with conscious breathing, we are reprogramming our body to no longer fall into this biochemical trap. Thus we lead happier and healthier lives and become more pleasant people to be around.

The ancient yoga scriptures inform us that we have a fixed amount of breaths allocated in our lifetime, so the slower and deeper they are, the longer we will live. Scientifically the idea of a set number of breaths is debatable, but the essence is true. And not only will the result be longevity, but the quality of the life you are living will increase through yoga practiced regularly, intelligently, and with an open heart.

Ujaii breathing with the application of *bandhas* and in conjunction with *vinyasa* is designed to generate heat from the core of the body. This heat is intensely purifying, and thus profuse sweating is common in beginners, but decreases very soon with regular practice. Even advanced practitioners who have intoxicated their body in some way will know about it, as yoga leaves no room for impurities; they will be expelled quickly and efficiently! Thus one is much more in touch with one's internal hygiene and automatically one's desires and cravings become more refined. Yoga never lies. If you have ingested, exposed yourself to, or put out impure materials, thoughts, or actions, these will manifest in your practice. Thus yoga is not an easy path, but a very effective and rewarding one. Furthermore, if you are fortunate enough to fall in love with asana, then *pranayama*, and eventually meditation practice, it will automatically inform your choices and invest your life with all the things that support a deeper connection to truth.

Ujaii pranayama means "victorious breath." It is a technique whereby, while breathing through the nose through a gentle contraction at the back of the throat, one lengthens, deepens, and sharpens the breath. It works hand in hand with the application of the *bandhas* or "locks." The three main *bandhas* are subtle internal muscular grips or holds that should remain gently engaged throughout the practice. In simple terms, *mula bandha*, or root lock, is achieved by squeezing the perineum and pulling up the pelvic floor. *Uddhiyana bandha* is the drawing back and up of the navel and a dropping of the tailbone. *Jalandhara bandha* is achieved by drawing the chin in, which results in the upper back broadening and shoulders releasing and ensures that the neck is protected and treated as an integral part of the spine. *Mula* and *jalandhara bandha* stimulate the parasympathetic nervous system, while *uddhiyana* stimulates the sympathetic nervous system. Thus the *bandha triyam*, or combination of these three main locks, also balances the nervous system. As the breath is slowly drawn deep into the body through *ujaii*, and the abdomen is being held back with *uddhiyana bandha*, the breath is instead directed into the thoracic ribcage all around, as well as the back of the body right down into the kidneys. On the slow and steady exhalation, the entire body experiences a release as the diaphragm, which is connected through fascia to the rest of the body, lifts. The skill to synchronize this internal movement with the external movement of the body is what is

referred to as *vinyasa*. (For a more detailed explanation, please refer to the *Sublimatio* section of Chapter 3.)

Increasingly, as the outward appearance of my asana practice becomes more impressive, I am asked the question, "But is it natural for the body to be able to do all that?" My reply is that yoga practice was never about being natural, as our "natural state" pertains to survival. Yoga is a practice that offers incredible levels of vitality, ultimately leading to the generation of supernatural powers. If the ego-mind manages not to get caught up with those, yoga is a path that leads to freedom, kaivalya.

Why a dynamic practice? Over the past twelve years, I have experimented with a variety of yoga styles and studied different schools of thought on the subject. In terms of combining health benefits, positive psychological effects, strengthening one's capacity to concentrate, and establishing a stream of consciousness that can be referred to as a dynamic form of meditation, I have found that a flowing *vinyasa* (breath-synchronized) practice is the most effective. Naturally there are times when a more static restorative or menstrual practice is more appropriate. To assist the practitioner in recognizing when this is the case, I established Quantum Assessment Methods.

OVERVIEW OF SUBTLE ANATOMY IN QUANTUM YOGA PRACTICE

PANCHAMAYA KOSHA

According to yoga philosophy, humans have five bodies, or layers, referred to as the *panchamaya kosha*. These are the physical body (*anamaya kosha*), the vital body (*pranamaya kosha*), the mental body (*manomaya kosha*), the consciousness body (*jnanamaya kosha*), and the bliss-body (*anandamaya kosha*).

The food body, or *anamaya kosha*, is the physical body. "You are what you eat," is a view that has been held in India since ancient times. Ayurveda in particular has explored this field and come up with holistic guidelines for healthy eating, furthermore, from a yoga point of view it is important that the food you ingest has been procured without causing undue harm to the environment or other sentient beings. Traditionally, this means a vegetarian diet and nowadays the focus is on food being organic and locally sourced.

PRANA

The material body is saturated with a subtle energy referred to as *prana*, which imbues it with life. In short, prana is that which gives life to matter. In the practice of yoga, we use the physical body to access and manipulate the vital body or *pranamaya kosha*. The system of the *bandhas*, or "locks," (subtle internal muscular grips or holds) represents a physiological support system for the body, but also a method whereby the prana (vital life force) is harnessed, directed, and centrally concentrated to flow upwards. Particularly in a dynamic practice, which involves jumping and thus impact to the body, this internal muscular engagement also protects from injury.

NADIS

The vital life force, or prana, taken in primarily through the breath, flows along 72,000 *nadis* (literally "rivers"), or channels, in the body. Of those, there are three main *nadis*. Hatha Yoga, which encompasses all physical practices of yoga, has as its primary objective to bring prana into *sushumna* ("ray of light") *nadi*, the central energy channel that runs along the spine. As the spine is our central structural support, its agility and alignment is therefore of utmost energetic importance. Balance is the key in this process. Thus *ida*, the moon channel that starts in the left nostril and flows down to the right big toe, and *pingala*, the sun channel that starts in the right nostril and flows down to the left big toe, are constantly being equalized. Once this state of perfect balance is achieved, prana automatically gathers in *sushumna nadi*.

CHAKRAS

Ida and *pingala* start at left and right nostril respectively and then crisscross through *sushumna* at six points, or chakras. These energy vortexes can be visualized as whirlpools where the prana gathers and spins, as its flow is concentrated where

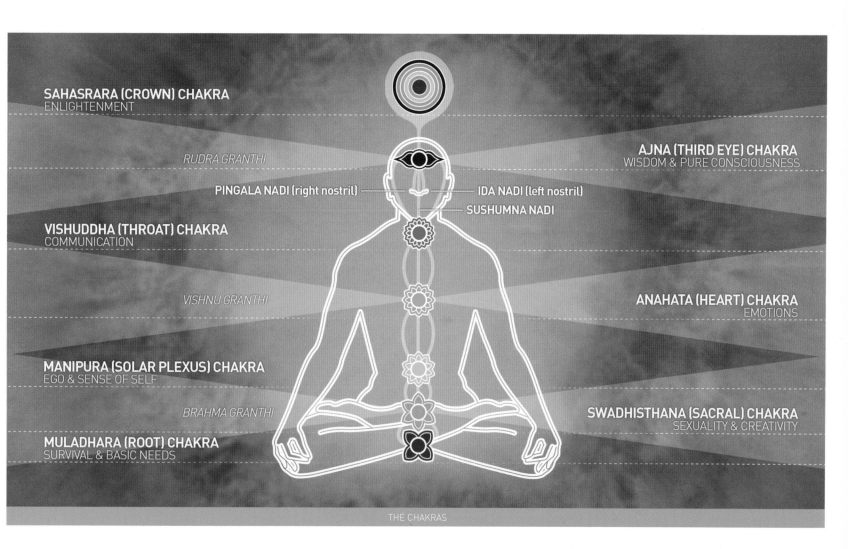

SAHASRARA (CROWN) CHAKRA
ENLIGHTENMENT

RUDRA GRANTHI

AJNA (THIRD EYE) CHAKRA
WISDOM & PURE CONSCIOUSNESS

PINGALA NADI (right nostril) —   — IDA NADI (left nostril)
                    SUSHUMNA NADI

VISHUDDHA (THROAT) CHAKRA
COMMUNICATION

VISHNU GRANTHI

ANAHATA (HEART) CHAKRA
EMOTIONS

MANIPURA (SOLAR PLEXUS) CHAKRA
EGO & SENSE OF SELF

BRAHMA GRANTHI

SWADHISTHANA (SACRAL) CHAKRA
SEXUALITY & CREATIVITY

MULADHARA (ROOT) CHAKRA
SURVIVAL & BASIC NEEDS

THE CHAKRAS

the main three rivers (*nadis*) cross. If the flow is inhibited at these points, it will manifest as an emotional disturbance, psychological imbalance, or disease. Of course, the opposite is also true, whereby such conditions will affect the flow.

Muladhara chakra is the "root" chakra located by the perineum and it relates to the level of consciousness concerned with survival and looking after one's basic needs. It is often visualized as red and its root sound, or *bija* mantra, is "*Lam.*" It relates to the sense of smell, controls the adrenal gland, and is of the earth element.

Swadhisthana means "her favorite abode" and is the sexual and creative center, located approximately three fingers below the navel. It is orange in color and the sound is "*Vam.*" It relates to the sense of taste, its element is water, and it controls the reproductive glands.

Manipura means "the jewel in the city" and this chakra is located at the solar plexus. This is the seat of the ego and gives the individual a sense of self. Its color is yellow and its *bija* mantra "*Ram.*" It relates to the sense of sight, its element is fire, and it is responsible for the pancreas and liver.

Anahata means "unstruck," referring to its vibrational aspect and the thus resulting sound being self-originated, i.e. unlike

conventional sound which is always the result of some sort of friction. It lies at the heart center and is our emotional core responsible for loving kindness and compassion. Its color is green, the sound "*Yam.*" It relates to the sense of touch and the element air and regulates the thymus gland responsible for the white blood cells and immune system.

Visuddhi, or "poison-free," is the throat chakra. It is responsible for communication and a harmonious interaction with the outer world. It allows for expression, sound, and speech. Its color is blue, its *bija* mantra "*Ham,*" and its element ether. It relates to the sense of hearing, and regulates the thyroid gland.

Ajna chakra is the "command center," as it is the seat of wisdom or Shiva, pure consciousness. Its *bija* mantra is "*Aum*" or "*Om*" and its color violet. It relates to the element akasha (subtle ether) and is responsible for the pineal gland.

KUNDALINI AND SHIVA-SHAKTI

With the application of the *bandhas* then, the balancing of *ida* and *pingala* and the harnessing of prana in sushumna, the thus strengthened upward flow of prana eventually awakens the mysterious kundalini shakti. This reservoir of psychic energy that lies dormant near our root is often represented as a three and a half coiled serpent goddess. Once unleashed, kundalini travels in spiralling movements up *sushumna nadi*. This Shakti (or power) meets Shiva (or higher consciousness) in the seat of wisdom at the third eye (*ajna chakra*) and this cosmic union engenders a transcendental shift in consciousness that causes the yogi to take a quantum leap towards a more liberated state of mind. The union of Shiva and Shakti are enjoyed beyond the physical confines of the body in the seventh, or crown chakra (**Sahasrara**), and people with psychic powers can see a radiant halo in enlightened beings. It is said that in this halo all the letters of the Sanskrit alphabet are to be found. Sahasrara can also be visualized as a thousand-petaled, multicolored lotus floating above the crown of the head. Its sound is the silent resonance of Om and it too pertains to the element akasha, or subtle ether.

VAYUS

The use of the term *prana* in general refers to a cosmic energy, and thus the individual's *pranamaya kosha* extends far beyond the boundaries of the physical body. In the context of the pranic effects and functions in the *anamaya kosha* however, we differentiate between five *vayus*, or winds. The element air is responsible for movement in the body and therefore the *vayus* describe these directional forces.

Prana vayu is the first, and provides ascent in the body, both in terms of physical lift of air and with it all tissues, as well

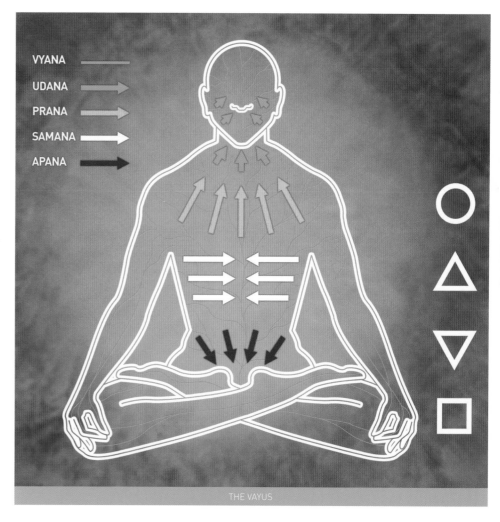

THE VAYUS

as engendering a rise in consciousness. It operates between the larynx and the top of the diaphragm and is responsible for respiration and speech.

Apana vayu, on the other hand, is responsible for elimination and thus operates below the navel moving downward. It gives the body the capacity for material creation.

Samana vayu is concentrated by the navel, moves back and forth sideways, and is responsible for digestion and the assimilation of nutrients from food.

Udana vayu is seated at the throat and above, moving upwards. It regulates swallowing, vomiting, and belching, but also activates the sensory organs of sight, smell, and hearing, as well as mental processes. It controls movement of the limbs and supports the erect posture of the body.

Vyana vayu flows throughout the body and thus ensures circulation of blood and lymph, and with it the supply of prana to all cells. It also acts as a pranic reserve force.

GRANTHIS

In our journey back towards union consciousness, the energetic ascent that we experience will encounter hindrances or psychic blocks that are referred to as granthis, or "knots." These were originally formed in our development as self-conscious individuals. Brahma *granthi* lies by *muladhara* chakra and pertains to our basic survival mechanisms, attachment to material things, and an excess of tamas. Vishnu *granthi* functions in the region of *anahata* chakra and is a result of emotional attachments and conditional love and manifests in high levels of *rajas*. Finally, *Rudra granthi* operates around *ajna* chakra and is caused by the identification with a self-limiting ego-identity and an attachment to *siddhis*. Through the conscious maintenance of the body (asana), control of the breath (*pranayama*), and application of the *bandhas*, these knots can be loosened. This is done by manipulation and reversal in the flow of the vayus.

BINDU

Bindu literally means "point". It is the potential for total implosion that we carry in the microcosm of our body. It is the spaceless void from whence we became manifest. This *bindu* is said to be located in our heads at the posterior fontanel near the pineal gland. Some Indian swamis, holy men, and other priestly types leave just a tuft of hair at the back of their heads to mark this point.

AMRIT (KECHARI MUDRA)

Tradition has it that from the *bindu* drops the sacred amrit, the nectar of immortality, a sort of vitality juice. This amrit drops unguarded down the body to eventually get consumed by the gastric fire. Thus we age. Many practices have been designed to harness this precious substance and stop it from being taken by flames. The most effective way, as repeatedly recommended in the Hatha Yoga Pradipika and other related scriptures, is through the application of *kechari* mudra. *Mudra* means "seal" and mudras are usually hand gestures that seal an attitude and set a certain energetic circuit in the body. Mudras work with the *nadis*, the pranic channels, and through their placement fix a specific energetic expression, like a temporary rewiring of cables. In the case of *kechari* mudra, the fixed position is that of the tongue being turned back in the mouth, so that the tip rests on the soft palate. With repeated practice, which can be done just sitting or combined with asana-pranayama, one can actually begin to taste the sweet milky amrit and trap it in the throat. Furthermore, the tongue is connected through a *nadi* to the root region and thus connects *muladhara* with *vissudhi* chakra. Ultimately *kechari* holds the potential to direct prana and thus further support the awakening of kundalini shakti.

THE MIND: JNANA, VIJNANA, AHANKARA, MANAS, CHITTA AND BUDDHI

When consciously refined through yoga practice, all these internal processes affect the human being on various levels. The manipulation of prana will have a direct impact on the physical well-being of the body, and it will also determine one's psychological state. The latter pertains to the third layer in the teaching of the five bodies, the *manomaya kosha*, or thought-body. This refers to cognition, inference, memory, imagination, and all mental activities. The mind in ancient India became the subject of great analysis and practical experimentation through yogic techniques. Jnana, or knowledge, results from experience. The sense objects are perceived through the organs of the senses and the thus resulting consciousness (*vijnana*) organizes this perception. It does so through the help of the ahankara that relates all experience back to the self. This basic dualistic modality then informs our patterns of thought (*chitta*) and the stuff that fills our mind (manas). A direct perception of truth is one that overcomes the limitations of the self, personal preference, and preconceived notions of reality, which pertain only to sense-perception and are limited by the ahankara, or "I-maker".

Thus this view on the functioning of the mind posits yet another organ, that of higher understanding referred to as the intellect, or *buddhi*. Here we enter another subtler layer of consciousness that constitutes the fourth body, or *vijnanamaya kosha*—the consciousness body. Although the buddhi still forms part of the experience of conceptual reality, it is also through the buddhi that we will be inspired to redirect out attention towards a nondual perception of reality, the object of which is the Atman, or higher self. Atman is our divine spark and is of the essence of Brahman, cosmic consciousness, the ultimate truth, or God. It is the same for everyone as the Atman is free from characteristics (the gunas); it is eternal and unchanging. Whereas thinking (*chitta*) has an object and an external subject, in yoga practice the subject is always internal. It is the self focused on the self, eliminating all that is not "real" in the ultimate sense of permanent and unconditioned. Thus with skillful practice consciousness is transformed and pierces through to a higher non-dual state that is of the nature of bliss. The ultimate body, or *anandamaya kosha*, is the bliss-body. It is infinite and all pervading.

At any point in time, we inhabit all five bodies. They are at our disposal and in our reach. It all depends on our level of consciousness. That which you are aware of is your reality. We have all been conditioned to accept just a very limited range of our potential for experience, never fully quenching our thirst for wisdom. Once you have found the path of yoga, you have come to the source, which lies within you. To access all five bodies with full awareness, the *sadhaka* (spiritual practitioner) must refine their state of being on all levels. This starts with our relationship to the outer world via the body, through the breath to our state of mind. Here we can turn the process around and transform that which we perceive as without from within.

THE QUANTUM SCIENCE OF SPIRITUALITY

When I first studied scriptures that described these esoteric principles and made promises of such metaphysical rewards, I interpreted them as being purely symbolic. To me, the kundalini stood for our psychological tendency to focus our concern on banal trivia ultimately pertaining to the ego-mind's need for self-preservation. Hence, it was stuck between *muladhara* (survival, basic needs) and *swadhisthana* (sexual and creative center) chakras. I thought this way until one day in Ibiza in 2002, when to my total surprise my kundalini really did stir. I'd had lots of problems with my joints at the time and felt like a doll whose hinges had come loose. I finally found myself in a situation where I had lots of time, and being in close rapport with nature, tucked away in the north of the island without a car, I was even more inclined for spiritual practice. I later also found out that the island is famed for its strong magnetic fields. Due to the condition of my body, I could not really do much asana practice, so I focused on *pranayama* and meditation. One evening, I suddenly felt an uncontrollable stirring within. I had to lie down and my body was writhing as though it were possessed by snakes. Spiraling tornados of energy seemed to be involuntarily rising from the tip of my limbs, but most concentrated from the root of the spine right up to the crown of the head. The sensation was incredibly pleasant but very frightening, as I had no control over it whatsoever. This is how the ancient manuals describe the release of kundalini shakti, the "serpent power," an energy that lies dormant at the base of the spinal column and when unleashed rises up the *sushumna nadi*, the central energy channel that runs along the spine. It repeated itself a few times over the following months and then stopped. I'd always written that type of experience off as the domain of the mystics and yet now I could no longer deny that it was real and profoundly transformative. Indeed my practice and life have never been the same since. Generally, I seem more constantly in touch with the primordial joy that lies at the very basis of existence. Of course I still get embroiled in a misidentification with the fluctuating reality all around me, but there seems to always be a very tangible part of me that knows, not just intellectually but right from my heart and gut, that all this is nothing compared to the wonder of being. After the initial experience, I felt like I had rediscovered a sort of lost innocence, the inner child having reclaimed its voice to reveal a unique kind of wisdom. My experience of nature became much more immediate and direct and at the same time my approach to life was marked by a new fearless open-mindedness that left more room for joy.

It so happened that at that same time, I had started reading a lot of books on quantum theories and these seemed to be speculating about things I was experiencing firsthand. I was astonished to discover that what these theories were describing on a macrocosmic level reflected the processes I was witnessing on the microcosmic level of the body. The division between particles and waves, energy and matter was becoming blurred. In fact, as those experiences unfolded I came to regard energy as much more substantial and real than matter could ever be. Just the way quantum mechanics introduced an unavoidable element of unpredictability or randomness into science, so these experiences were forcing me to re-evaluate yoga practice and philosophy. In my research, I encountered similar difficulties to those described by the physicists. This is when I first came across Heisenberg's Uncertainty Principle, which purports that it is not possible to measure the present state of the universe precisely, as the very act of measuring effects it. Similarly, the deeper my consciousness spread into the hidden recesses of my body, the faster it changed. I would detect areas of blockage and direct *prana*, only to discover that behind the tension and pain laid real storerooms of energy. Once a blockage in the body has been undone, a rush of energy is unleashed, much like a dam breaking in a river. And just as one has to be very cautious in doing away with dams, so the mind has to be ready to channel the energy when it comes, and have established the integrity and clarity to be able to cope with the emotional consequences. Blockages usually accrue over years of protecting oneself from the intensity and challenge of actually coming into one's power, of realizing the oneness of all.

These experiences are precious and rare, and one must hold deep gratitude for experiencing such grace. Although regular asana and especially *pranayama* and meditation practice will make them a lot more likely, there is no guarantee. You may spend the rest of your life diligently doing daily sadhana without any such energetic manifestations. Yet, you can be sure that the yoga practice will have increased the quality of your life in the right way. You will have benefited from better health, higher levels of vitality, and a generally more peaceful and relaxed disposition. Perhaps kundalini shakti is shy and taking her time, winding her way up *sushumna nadi* slowly and unnoticed and enjoying her quiet journey.

AYURVEDA: THE SCIENCE OF LIFE

Veda means "knowledge." The most ancient of the Vedas, the Rigveda, is a collection of mantras that alludes to the juxtaposition between the macrocosm of the universe and the microcosm of the human body. In the four Upavedas, or "secondary Vedas," this concept is further explored. The Dhanurveda pertains mainly to the practice of martial arts. It is here that the science of the *marma* points, or "energy junctions," in the body, which are also used in Ayurvedic massage and yoga practice, is explained in detail. The Ayurveda reveals medicine for body and mind. Music, dance, and literature form the theme for the Gandharva Veda, while the Sthapatya Veda discloses the secrets of *vastu*, or the directional influences and how these inform architecture.

Much of Ayurvedic knowledge was lost over time, but in recent years this ancient system of medicine has experienced a resurgence in popularity, as people realize that its holistic methodology often achieves deeper effects than conventional medicine and thus yields long term results. Ayurveda's approach is initially preventative rather than curative. It shows a person how to live in harmony with one's own nature, as well as the natural cycles of the day, the seasons, and life. As the science of Ayurveda and yoga sprang from the same fountain, they complement each other. They are based on the same worldview, except that one focuses on life, the other on transcendence. Again, it is generally accepted by all spiritual

traditions that in order to get beyond something, you must first embrace and master that thing. An understanding of Ayurveda will lead to this mastery of life (ayu) and all things pertaining to this world. Quantum Yoga encourages you to recognise things as they truly are and consciously manifest this truth in all your actions.

Ayurveda views the world as made up of five elements, the *pancha mahabhuta*. From gross to subtle, these are earth (*prthivi*), water (*ap*), fire (*tejas*), air (*vayu*), and ether (*akasha*). Water (cold) and fire (hot) interact with air to form the *doshas* (biological humors). The *doshas* operate to keep harmony between the elements in the body and ensure the functioning of the body's systems. Each person holds all three *doshas*, but in varying distributions. One's prakriti (personal doshic distribution) is determined at birth. Prakriti turns into *vrkirti* when *dosha* imbalances set in due to improper lifestyle. If one's yoga practice is constructed in a manner that takes into account one's prakriti, as well as the effect that such things as season, age, circumstances, and emotional state will have on one's internal balance, it will lead to the ideal state where the body-mind is at perfect ease.

The *doshas* are the main factors in Ayurvedic thought, as they represent the underlying forces in the workings of both body and mind. Through the interplay of the gunas, the five elements, when imbued with *prana*, manifest as the *doshas* (biological temperaments) in sentient beings.

Unless they are tridoshic, meaning their *doshas* are in a perfect state of balance, people either tend very much towards one *dosha*, or two *doshas* as the dominant forces. It is important to understand, though, that even if you have a prevalence of a certain *dosha* or two, a disturbance may manifest in any of the *doshas*, depending on circumstance and change your particular *doshic* state. Also, the natural tendency of most people is to be drawn to those things that reinforce one's doshic condition. So for example, if you are a fiery person, you are bound to like coffee and spicy foods.

Vata is the *dosha* of air and thus is responsible for movement. It is dry, volatile, cold, irregular, and flighty. A person who has a predominance of *vata* will usually be thin, with dry skin, frizzy hair, hard but brittle nails, and uneven teeth, and the eyes may have a grayish tinge. *Vata* people have great ideas, good short-term memory, and are often impulsive, but lack the stamina and discipline to go through with things. A disturbance in *vata* is usually brought about by unstable circumstances, windy conditions, and upheaval or change in general. It is exacerbated by raw foods, marijuana and psychedelic drugs, and a lack of routine.

Pitta is the dosha of fire and a degree of water, and is responsible for digestion. It is hot, passionate, and active. *Pitta*-types have reddish, irritable skin, and tend to sweat profusely. They are of medium and muscular build, their hair is often thin and straight and grays early, their nails are rubbery, eyes sharp, and the teeth tend to yellow and the gums bleed easily. *Pitta* people have fiery temperaments and like to make things happen. Their memory is astute, their sex drive high, and anger a predominant emotion. *Pitta* is exacerbated by spicy foods, stimulants, and hot conditions.

Kapha is the dosha of earth and water, and is thus responsible for grounding. *Kapha*-types are usually heavyset with oily, thick, wavy hair, big soft eyes, thick skin, and large, strong teeth and nails. They are of a mild, often lazy disposition, but once set into motion, have great stamina. They have good long-term memory, avoid confrontation, and are often quite reserved. *Kapha* is exacerbated by oily, stodgy foods and alcohol, a sedentary lifestyle, and a lack of stimulation or exposure to the outdoors.

Food is regarded as extremely important in Ayurveda, as once consumed by the digestive fire, it nourishes one *dhatu* after the next in a chain. The *dhatus* are the basic bodily tissues or constituents of the human body. The seven dhatus are:

THE SEVEN DHATUS		ELEMENT
RASA	FLUIDS, HORMONES, AND LYMPHS	WATER
RAKTA	BLOOD	FIRE
MAMSA	FLESH, MUSCLES, AND CUTIS	EARTH
MEDHA	FAT	WATER AND EARTH
ASTHI	BONES AND TEETH	AIR AND ETHER
MAJJA	MARROW	FIRE
SHUKRA	SEMEN (OJAS), THE SUBLIMATED FORM OF SEXUAL ENERGY AND OVUM (ARTAVA)	WATER

Rasa is the first to receive the food's nutrients and *shukra/arthava* the last. Ayurveda tends to treat most things in terms of the *dhatus* partly because they indicate how far down the chain a problem has advanced and also reveal which *dosha* is out of whack. There are many vata disorders; as they are usually acute the cure is thus relatively straightforward. There are far fewer kapha disorders, but as they take time to form, they tend to be harder to cure.

Like yoga, Ayurveda recognizes that the ideal and indeed natural state of the human being is when the body is at perfect ease. So how can we avoid the onset of disease in the first place? How can we apply Ayurveda's holistic approach and its teaching of the *doshas* (biological humors) to our understanding of the Assessment Methods of Quantum Yoga?

In yoga, just as in our choice of food and lifestyle, we need to recognize that individuals tend to be attracted to those things and activities that reinforce their natural tendencies and therefore cause further imbalance. Again, to use the more straightforward example of food, while salad and raw foods may be regarded as good for your health, these light foods only exacerbate ungrounded, spacey, and windy feelings (which can manifest both emotionally and physically) in someone who is a vata-type or whose vata is disturbed by recent upheaval. Yet, most people who are in that flighty state tend to pick at light foods on irregular occasions and usually while distracted with things other than eating. Similarly, *kapha*-types or those whose *kapha* is imbalanced due to consumption, boredom, or depression, which manifests as laziness, sloth, and torpor, would do well to snack on a few carrot sticks, but more likely opt for oily foods like crisps or chips.

And so in the choice of yoga practice. The air—or *vata*—types are in their comfort zone when they literally feel like they are floating. So any practice that will inspire imagination and induce a trancelike state will attract them. Remember that we are trying to find a practice that brings out the best in us, while keeping us stimulated. As such, I am not suggesting that a *vata*-type should instead put themselves through an austere routine of grounding and strengthening poses, especially because they will not stick with that for long. When *vata* is excessive or imbalanced, the ideal yoga practice is one that satisfies this need for lightness and motion, and yet only yields concrete and satisfying results through a solid understanding of gravity and a firm connection to Mother Earth.

I have deliberately named the "Birds" sequence, which contains many postures that emulate various types of birds, after our flighty, winged friends. These postures specifically give you a small or unusual surface area to balance on, to encourage you to exploit the upward pranic force of lightness. Yet this can only be done if the body surface that is in contact with the ground maximizes its connection. This capacity to firmly connect to the earth, distributing the weight in a balanced manner, is also referred to as bandha, or lock. The whole flavor of the "Birds" sequence is thus one of embracing gravity in order to master it. For a *vata*-type, or in times when *vata* is upset, the yogi does need to ground and strengthen, commit to a pose, and use slow, deep *ujaii* breathing to increase inner heat, focus the mind, and still the emotions. Of course to a degree this goes for all yoga practice, but vata in particular benefits from these practices as it is responsible for inner turbulence.

Pitta-types want to see results from their actions, so they will tend to go for the more dynamic, challenging yoga routines.

When *pitta* is disturbed, your natural tendency will be to want to thrash it out on the mat. This aggressive energy however is what often causes, if not injury, a depletion of energy that will leave the yogi sweaty and exhausted at the end of practice. Although burning through this passionate need for stimulation and achievement may grant short-term satisfaction, ultimately this is not what will bring about the state of clarity and ease that paves the way for lasting inner peace. It is very hard for a *pitta*-type to pull the reins on this need to expend energy, so in the "Heroes" Sequence, the practice is still suitably challenging, but the energy is expended evenly like butter on toast. Furthermore, when this pushy *pitta* energy prevails, the person is usually only aware of the more obvious sensations. To encourage subtle perception, such as that of sound vibration, but still allow the *pitta*-type to feel satisfied that they are working hard, the Heroes sequence puts the yogi into horse-riding stance and there has them chant the *bija* mantras while visualizing the chakras.

The Heroes theme, which implies achievement through courageous struggle, is appealing to a *pitta*-type. The practitioner will soon come to realize, however, that the more tricky parts of the sequence are best mastered through a softer, more receptive approach that flows with momentum, understands the laws of physics, and allows for a clever and conscious use of prana. The ego-mind is thus held in check. There are many variations on the Hero's Pose

(*Virasana*), which, unless there is an already existing injury, contributes to the safeguarding of the knees, which typically suffer in a *pitta* person.

So, to regulate *pitta*, we must find a practice that will control and channel this forceful energy. Just as in tantra, the energetic flow of the passions are reverted upward towards higher consciousness, rather than suppressed or directed outwards towards sense satisfaction, so here we do not want to end up frustrated by the superficial imposition of a softer approach. Rather, we offer this yogi powerful alternatives to the more obvious ways of applying oneself in spiritual practice—ways that result in true transformation. The challenge is to keep channeling the energy in the right direction, expending it evenly and always remaining receptive and gentle.

Kapha-types do not like change, especially when repeated and sudden. They will be attracted by the slower and gentler styles of yoga. They do not lack focus, nor are they weak, but they are not particularly open to getting spontaneously excited about something. When *kapha* is imbalanced, there may even be a preference for seated meditation practice over asana. This is the time however that the body should be encouraged to move dynamically. The system needs to be awakened and the inner energetic flow kick-started.

Muladhara chakra is the seat of earthly concerns pertaining to basic survival. The energy here tends to move down and make a person feel heavy, stagnant, and worried. Therefore, above all in regulating *kapha*, *mula bandha* needs to be strengthened and encouraged. All variations on *Vajrasana* (Diamond-Thunderbolt Pose), which is done on the tips of the toes, will entice a pulling up on the physical as well as the subtle energetic level, which automatically also lifts the spirits.

The Lotus Mandala is thus the most dynamic of the sequences, and contains many stimulating poses. For example, the dynamic inversions such as the Handstand (*Adho Mukha Vrikshasana*) and the Forearm Balance (*Pincha Mayurasana*), which I often call the double espresso of asana practice, really cause a very tangible invigoration. On top of particularly benefitting from these poses, *kapha*-types are actually often in a good position to master them, as their strength and focus are essential. To avoid injury though, this group of asana does require careful preparation, and thus the Sublimatio ensures spinal awakening and pelvic stability. *Kapha* people often have good stamina and once the momentum has been gathered to move, these earth-water types can go on for a long time. The art lies therefore in getting the ball rolling safely.

THE QUANTUM ASSESSMENT METHODS

In assessing what the ideal practice is for you on a particular day, consider first of all the practicalities of time and space. If you are not practicing on a stable surface, you may need to keep your center of gravity lower and prioritize horse-riding stance variations over *Suryanamaskara* (Sun Salutations), and floor work over standing poses. If you are stuck in a corridor, you will have to construct your sequence on a linear plane, which can be useful in supporting your understanding of the geometry of poses. If you have very little time, you may want to limit the Sublimatio to an internal journey of the mind's eye from feet to crown in *Tadasana* (Mountain Pose), and weave the standing sequence into the dynamic flow.

Next you want to take into account the season and time of day. The colder it is, the more you need to build and sustain heat. If it is very hot, on the other hand, you may want to use this opportunity to work more deeply into the stretches. In the morning, you want to awaken the system and set yourself up for a constructive day. Take into account that *kapha* (mucus) prevails in the morning and the system thus needs to be cleansed through vigorous *pranayama* and asana such as twists and backbends that support the body's capacity to eliminate. Daytime practice must take into account the prevalence of *pitta* (bile) and thus focus on applying the body in a balanced manner while centering the mind. In the afternoon vata sets in, so strengthening and grounding exercises are

key. In the evening, you need to process the events of the day and come to a state of deep stillness and relaxation. Any disturbance in *vata* (wind) will engender restlessness. Thus to ensure good sleep, one should finish with long-held stilling poses such as *Paschimottanasana* (Forward-Bend) and *Sarvangasana* (Shoulderstand) variations.

Most importantly, take into consideration your personal type and how circumstances may be affecting you that day. If there are injuries, you need to stabilize these vulnerable areas in the Sublimatio and avoid any postures that will aggravate the condition. Should there be disease on an organic level, you need to integrate postures that strengthen the affected functions and make sure not to deplete the system as a whole.

If *vata* (air) prevails, you need to focus on grounding and strengthening. Excess *vata* makes it difficult to concentrate; one feels spacey and often anxious. You may be a *vata*-type or an imbalance in this field may just be a result of unsettling circumstances, such as a move, a trip, a break-up, or even just a windy day. The extremities often feel cold, and special attention should be paid to safeguarding ankles and wrists. Standing balances and any postures that posit an altered foundation and therefore challenge one's relationship with gravity are very useful. The breath is often shallow and needs to be deepened and lengthened through such *pranayama* practices as *nadi shodana*.

Prevalence in *pitta* (fire-water) manifests as an excess in heat in the body-mind. You may be feeling hot-tempered, hyperactive, and angry, or the body may feel tense and restless. This energy needs to be harnessed and channelled. The focus in a *pitta*-regulating practice is on expending the energy evenly and awakening one's capacity to fine-tune the senses. Impatience and pushiness can lead to injury and a feeling of depletion after the body has been "punished" through excessively vigorous practice. The practitioner needs to realise that being kind to oneself does not mean slacking, but rather directing the effort toward refinement of movement, which ensures correct alignment and smooth transitions. The exhalation is often much stronger and longer than the inhalation and therefore the inhalation needs to be supported and made conscious through such *pranayama* practices as *viloma* or *bhastrika* with *antara kumbhaka*. (See Chapter 5.)

Imbalance in *kapha* (earth-water) manifests through sloth, torpor, and a lazy feeling of heaviness. Before vigorously kick-starting the body in the dynamic flow, make sure to prepare by bringing the awareness to the feet, strengthening the core, and ensuring pelvic stability. *Kapha*-types often hold tension in the hips and thus supporting the body's ability to safely open up this region is especially important. Any arm-balancing inversions and backbends are intensely invigorating and

thus very useful. To keep things moving is the main motto here. The inhalation is often longer than the exhalation. Thus the capacity to release and let go on the exhale needs to be supported through such *pranayama* practices as *bandha triyam* in *bhaya kumbhaka*. (See Chapter 5.)

Remember that all three *doshas* always coexist and that the most important aspect of your yoga practice is ensuring a state of balance. Cultivating deep awareness and responding intuitively to the feedback that you are getting during your practice is key in supporting an interactive approach. You may for example have set out to do an awakening and invigorating practice, but then realize that actually grounding and strengthening is more important on that day. Quantum Yoga is a journey in self-healing, creative expression, and the art of receptivity. As soon as consciousness spreads deeper into your body, it will begin to transform, which will in turn affect consciousness. Using the Quantum Grouping and Sequencing laws explained below, you will be able to direct this ongoing dynamic towards self-realization.

Setting an intention for your practice is a great way of putting your personal experience into a wider context. I often use the sacred ancient mantra: *Loka Samastha Suki No Bhavantu* (May All Beings Everywhere be Happy and Free) and often dedicate my practice to another person, plant, animal, or an idea. When confronted with unpleasant sensations and the self-limiting thoughts these often cause, bringing myself back to the initial intention puts these into perspective. Higher intention in spiritual practice represents a sort of intelligent selflessness that ends up helping you to stick with it. Intention alone however does not suffice and skillful means and disciplined application are equally as important. How often were your intentions good, but the outcome nevertheless negative? Therefore, one must pay attention to what is really going on and be careful not to impose an idealistic vision in an inappropriate way. One should study universal principles and guidelines and learn how to apply them to one's own life.

Here are a few charts that will further your understanding of how to assess your ideal yoga practice using the system of Ayurveda[9]. Each of the three doshas has a certain character that determines the substances consumed by the body, every action performed, and every thought generated by the mind.

DOSHA SEATS IN THE BODY

It is to be understood that all *doshas* are present all over the body and a particular *dosha* may predominate in some regions more than others. *Kapha* houses itself primarily from the head to the chest region, *pitta* from chest to navel, and *vata* from the navel to the feet. All movements are due to *vata*, all metabolic transformations occur because of *pitta*, and *kapha* is responsible for lubrication and stability. As the brain is composed of fat, it is hence *kapha*.

TYPICAL DOSHA CHARACTERISTICS

VATA	PITTA	KAPHA
DRY	OILY	OILY
COLD	HOT	COLD
LIGHT	LIGHT	HEAVY
IRREGULAR	INTENSE	STABLE
MOBILE	FLUID	VISCOUS
ROUGH	LIQUID	SMOOTH

THE RELATION OF DOSHAS WITH THE TIMES OF DAY, AGE AND PHASES OF DIGESTION[10]

	KAPHA	PITTA	VATA
DAYTIME	MORNING (06.00 - 10.00)	MIDDAY (10.00 - 14.00)	EVENING (14.00 - 18.00)
NIGHTTIME	EARLY NIGHT (18.00 - 22.00)	MIDNIGHT (22.00 - 02.00)	LATE NIGHT (02.00 - 06.00)
AGE	CHILDHOOD	YOUTH	OLD AGE
DIGESTION	INITIAL STAGE OF DIGESTION	MIDDLE STAGE OF DIGESTION	LAST STAGE OF DIGESTION

RELATIONSHIP BETWEEN DOSHAS AND SEASONS[11]

	LATE WINTER	SPRING	SUMMER	RAIN	AUTUMN	EARLY WINTER
VATA			ACCUMULATION	AGGRAVATION	NORMALCY	
PITTA				ACCUMULATION	AGGRAVATION	NORMALCY
KAPHA	ACCUMULATION	AGGRAVATION	NORMALCY			

PART TWO

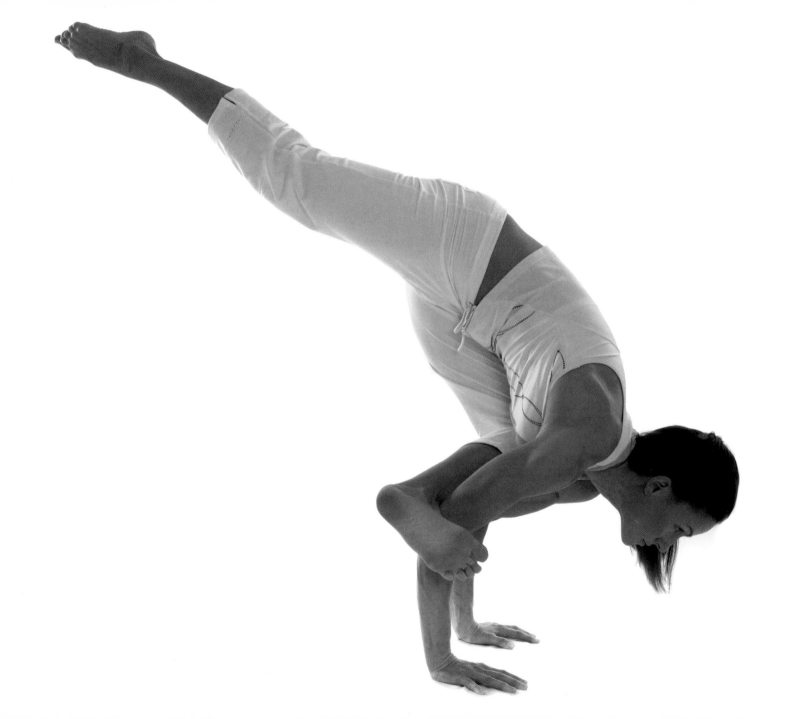

CHAPTER THREE
THE QUANTUM YOGA GROUPING AND SEQUENCING LAWS

A Quantum Yoga sequence is constructed like a musical symphony. It begins with a gentle introduction, to fine-tune the ear and awaken the consciousness to the unfolding of greater physical sensation. It rapidly picks up in pace, and then plateaus at a sustainable level of intensity. Here we prepare for the peak pose, which constitutes the apex of the sequence. Thereafter, if certain body parts need to be counterstretched or muscle groups strengthened to balance the intensity of the peak pose, this will also be factored in. Then commences the finishing sequence, which usually integrates focusing and grounding inversions that energetically consolidates the practice. There should be a pose that clearly marks the end of the practice and sets the yogi up for Savasana, the total state of surrender and relaxation, where all is still.

SUSTAINING THE FLOW AND LINKING

Classically, asana are linked dynamically through half or full *vinyasas*, which refer to the *Chaturanga Dandasana* (Four-Limbed Staff, or Press-Up Pose, often shortened to *Chatwari*), Upward-Facing Dog, and Downward-Facing Dog movements that also form part of the Sun Salutations. However, there are many other ways of linking asana dynamically. Part of spontaneous creation is to allow one asana to inform the next and listen for the body's impulses and needs to move into certain areas that require opening or strengthening.

In this way, one may only need to make subtle shifts in positioning to move from one posture to the next. If a set of poses has to be done on both sides, it is imperative to remember the sequence of asana one has done on the first side. This forms part of the cultivation of dharana, our faculty for concentration. The second side can either be done in the same order or working backwards, such as in the Birds Floor Work section. Flowing in this manner also highlights the subtle differences in poses that in their outward form would appear very similar. The subtle shift you have to make to flow from one asana into a structurally similar one will bring to your awareness the pose's essential form and unique energetic effect.

TIMINGS

How many breaths you chose to hold your postures for depends entirely on your needs that day, as well as how much time you have in total. Styles such as Ashtanga, where all postures apart from the finishing are held for five breaths, propagate a fixed number of breaths. In Quantum Yoga, you are encouraged to choose. If you are regulating *vata*, a fixed number of breaths can help control the flighty tendency and the postures should be held a little longer where possible. Where *pitta* is imbalanced, we need to be focusing on consistent expenditure of energy. In other words, take yourself out of the pose as soon as that forceful tendency manifests, and focus on refining the transitions between poses, so that you end up with a smooth flow. Where *kapha* prevails, the postures do not need to be held for too long. Keeping it dynamic and moving is the key, while of course ensuring safety through *bandhas* and correct alignment.

In the spirit of balance, when it comes to postures that are done on each side, we need to ensure an even breath-count. However, if an imbalance already exists, you may choose to deliberately hold the weaker or stiffer side longer. The more you practice with the level of awareness that Quantum Yoga cultivates, the faster you'll be able to intuitively sense the correct length to remain in postures. This of course does *not* mean just doing what is easy or comes naturally, but rather doing what you have learned to recognize as best for you at the time, which is often exactly the opposite of what feels easy or natural.

LEADING WITH LEFT OR RIGHT

In most traditional yoga sequences, the student is directed to lead each asana with the right side of the body. Quantum Yoga encourages you to vary. In my experience, the practitioner pays greater attention to the first side they work on, and tends to therefore hold it for a longer time. Unless you are left-handed or have been injured on the right, the left side is for most of us the awkward side. As we pay more attention

to the first side we carry out, it is therefore a good idea to sometimes allow this awkward side to take the lead. This may not result in you being ambidextrous, but it will certainly heighten your awareness and also unconsciously leave you open to approaching situations other than in the obvious and conditioned way. We live in a society that is mostly left-brain orientated, where typically right-brained processes such as intuition, creativity, and what is traditionally regarded as the "feminine" manner of feeling your way into situations is not encouraged. In yoga, however, you are not under pressure, nor are you competing against anyone, so allow for a softer approach and sometimes let the weaker side of your body reveal new ways of moving.

USE OF PROPS

Certain styles of yoga, such as Iyengar Yoga, have made the use of props into a fine art. Indeed raising or supporting certain parts of the body can lead to a widening range of movement. For a certain muscle to fire up or release, you often need to restrict movement of another set of muscles. The body has habitual ways of functioning. Often we unconsciously compensate for weaknesses and avoid stiff areas in order not to experience unpleasant feelings. At the same time, in our practice there may be a tendency to just go for the obvious sensations, thinking we are only doing the posture correctly if it really hurts and the outer form looks

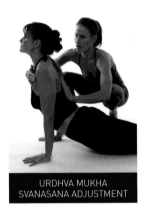

URDHVA MUKHA
SVANASANA ADJUSTMENT

about right. To get into the more unusual areas of the body, it is important to understand the essence of the pose. This often means taking a step back and simplifying the pose or using the aid of props. However, props should only be used where necessary to avoid reliance on outer supports. Ideally the yogi should cultivate a practice that can be done anytime and anywhere. Otherwise, the mind that anyway has a tendency to procrastinate will have yet another reason to convince you not to do your practice. For Quantum Yoga you only need to do one thing: start. The rest will unfold.

ADJUSTMENTS

Styles such as Ashtanga Vinyasa lay great claim to the benefit of adjustments. These can of course be useful, but should never push the body beyond its limits. I know from my own experience that one bad adjustment can lead to years of dealing with the injuries that result. Good adjustments simply encourage the body to open to its full capacity. Only ever adjust poses that you have experience with! When adjusting, one must get away from an idea of the "correct" outer form of the asana and embrace the essence of the pose. What is this pose meant to be doing for the practitioner? We are not hammering round screws into square holes. If you are adjusting, cultivate the kind of compassionate vision that can see where the energy flow is blocked and be motivated to awaken the other person's capacity to move beyond.

Recognize when your tendency to impose an ideal view onto a real body manifests, and replace it with the attitude that you are investigating how the asana can better serve this individual. Finally, cultivate teamwork when adjusting students or friends and encourage verbal feedback.

An actual outline of adjustment techniques goes beyond the scope of this book, but the following are a couple of useful general pointers. Go in slowly! Remember that you are entering someone's personal space and they may not be used to being touched. Once you have laid hands on the practitioner, do so with the full palm and without hesitation. Feeble adjustments from the tips of the fingers can feel creepy, unless you are simply pointing out a part of the body where pure verbal doesn't suffice. To adjust with confidence you need to be stable on your feet. Cultivate a firm connection to the ground and keep your center of gravity low. Breathe with the yogi you are adjusting. Although you don't want to impose your breath rate on them, a steady, powerful quality of breath will inspire depth and calm. Do not tug at the person's extremities! Identify the root of the movement; the closer you can get to it, the better. Joints are generally the most vulnerable parts. Respect the integrity of the joint and ligaments while stretching the muscles. Remember that any stretch goes two ways. As you encourage one direction, you need to make sure that the other side, which often forms the foundation of the pose, does not give way. Hereby you will avoid taking the yogi off balance. Nevertheless, always stand or sit in a manner where you are sure to catch them if they fall. Also, after you've adjusted someone, move away slowly, as the person will often topple as soon as you do. The reason is not merely because they may have been leaning on you. You constitute a magnetic field and as you draw away, the body you've been close to will feel that shift. Finally, keep an eye on your friend's facial expression, as this, along with the sound of their breath, communicates directly whether or not you are pushing them too far. As an experienced teacher, you can gradually be firmer with students. Once you can recognize when they are simply panicking, you will be able to take them beyond what are primarily psychological restrictions and lack of self-confidence or physical experience.

PAIN

There is no such thing as good pain. Short, sharp, sudden jolts of pain in particular are a clear way of your body telling you to back off, and you should heed this signal. Discomfort, unusual sensations, and unexpected feelings that accompany the widening of your range of movement are the building blocks of all Hatha Yoga. By practicing asana, you train your capacity to remain steady and at ease in all situations, be they physical, emotional, or transcendental. The main reason to keep adding more difficult postures to your Quantum practice

as you advance, is to keep training this skill. If it becomes too easy, you will not pay attention. You are deliberately taking yourself outside of your comfort zone. Naturally there are times when a nurturing or restorative practice is more appropriate, but those should be rendered relatively rare as you grow stronger through regular practice.

Why do injuries happen? Apart from being badly adjusted, I believe that the reason for self-inflicted injuries is twofold: ego and lack of attention. The Quantum Method has been developed to avoid both. If you are designing and choosing your sequence as you go along in answer to the impulses your body is sending you, you can't but pay attention. In this way, not only are you tapping into your power to manifest your own reality, but you are also avoiding disrespecting your body's signals by blindly pushing through a one-size-fits-all prefabricated sequence. When following a sequence you have been given, the ego's desire to master it awakens. This is not a bad thing and it's rooted in the fact that we all want recognition and have been conditioned to only feel worthy if we perform well. So if we go right to the root of wanting to feel loved and express that love in the most direct possible way by investigating our own needs and actively providing solutions, this leaves little space for the self-denying and destructive part of the ego.

Another important aspect to mention here is heat. In my experience, asana practice that lacks *vinyasa* coupled with *ujaii* breathing and *bandhas* does not protect the yogi adequately from injury. If strict attention is paid to structure and alignment such as in Iyengar Yoga, this represents a possible alternative to working with inner heat and core control. Many styles outside the Krishnamacharya lineage, much as I respect their holistic approach to yoga in general, in my experience take their students into quite advanced poses without sufficient preparation, attention to breath or inner muscular engagement, or much instruction pertaining to correct alignment. You can of course get around the problem of inner heat by putting your students into sauna-like conditions, but this does not allow for independent practice and the freedom that comes with it. More importantly, it ultimately reduces the body's capacity to generate inner heat, which purifies the system much more deeply than repeatedly sweating through the same set sequence in artificial conditions.

CLASSIFICATION OF ASANA ACCORDING TO PHYSIOLOGICAL EXPRESSION AND ENERGETIC EFFECT

When grouping asana, we need to take into account the fact that they can be classed either by *type*, (i.e., standing pose, backbend, inversion, etc.) or *effect*, (i.e., energizing, stilling, focusing, etc.) In the Quantum Yoga Grouping and Sequencing system, we start with the outer form in order to sustain coherence in movement, but bear in mind that we are orchestrating a sequence that reflects an energetic flow, which is in accord with the particular effect we are planning to achieve. Most asana belong to several groups, as they work into various parts of the body and can also have very different effects depending on what their placement is in the sequence and how long they are held. In the photo charts following each grouping section of this chapter, I have chosen to display those postures that would be typically practiced at this stage of a Quantum Yoga sequence. So for example, the posture on the cover of this book, the full *Shiva Natarajasana*, or dancing Shiva, is a standing balance pose, but also a backbend. I have placed the less challenging versions of this pose in the Standing Balance section, but the full posture in the later Backbends section, as most yogis need to have done quite a bit of preparation to take their body into this beautiful but challenging asana safely. Also remember that there exists an endless array of asana, so please feel free to use other postures that you are familiar with in the appropriate sections.

In terms of time allocated to the various groupings, with regard to the respective *dosha* one has chosen to focus on regulating, I hesitated to put together a chart like the one below. I work best intuitively, and I would encourage you to do so, too. To hone intuition, though, one requires experience, which can be more effective with some guidance. Also in a flowing practice—especially as the yogi becomes more advanced and is still able to sustain an overall harmonic energy curve even within varying complex compositions—the groups need not be so clearly demarcated.

HOW OFTEN SHOULD I PRACTICE?

With yoga practice, as with most things, it is much more advisable to do a little bit daily than to go for the occasional full-on yoga workout. Yoga is spiritual hygiene and thus should become as natural to you as brushing your teeth. If you are the type of person who tends to really go for a powerful asana practice every time you hit the mat, then I do think that taking a day or even an entire weekend off gives your body a chance to assimilate the expansion that your practice will have brought. It is best if on those days you can still keep up the meditation and *pranayama*. If you train yourself in measure, you will avoid any future problems with addictions. If addiction is already there, replacing it with an attachment to asana-*pranayama* is a good idea to begin with, but with time again please try to cultivate a healthier approach to it!

Another phenomenon I often see in students is that they are motivated by guilt. It is my hope that through the Quantum approach, yoga will become something that we do because the body-mind's intelligence longs for it. We deserve to feel our best.

At any rate, to be truly successful with yoga, you absolutely must find time daily to dissociate from outer reality and allow yourself to just be with the breath. This can even be done in a crowd of people if necessary, though a more convenient moment is ideal. After a period of daily disciplining yourself to dissociate in this way, it will become natural and even enjoyable to you.

Just a word of warning here, in order to avoid any misunderstanding: yoga is *not* about spacing or dropping out! It should make you more alert, stronger, and a competent and kind addition to the society you have chosen to be part of. Naturally, the tradition of renunciation also factors strongly in yoga culture, but consciously renouncing something means that you have mastered it first!

The most common excuse your mind will throw out for not doing your practice is that you simply haven't got the time. As Danny Paradise always smilingly points out to his students, "Yoga adds about twenty years onto your life, so it doesn't take time, it gives time!" Not only that, the quality of that life increases massively. Danny bases his opinion not only on his own experience, but on his close rapport with Western yogis who have practiced yoga since the 1960s and are now at an age that is associated with deterioration. Yet these individuals continue to refine their practice and live active and joyful lives that most people in their twenties and thirties barely match up to.

FOOD

Not only is it more enjoyable, but also energetically a lot more potent to practice on an empty stomach. Generally, it is advisable to avoid eating or drinking anything for one hour before asana practice. Heavier food, depending on your metabolic rate, can take much longer to digest. However, do not let the fact that you have eaten or drunk something relatively recently, or that you need to snack on something light because you are hungry, put you off from practicing. As a yoga teacher cycling about town, there are days when, if I stuck to the one-hour rule, I'd never eat!

THE QUALITY OF YOUR PRACTICE

I think by this time it should be pretty clear to most readers that yoga is not about mastering fancy postures. The main reason to keep challenging oneself with new and more difficult asana, apart from direct health benefits, is to train the mind. Therefore, if you are at the stage in which a very basic asana practice is difficult, this does not mean that your practice is any less valid than another. I remember encountering a saddhu in Rishikesh, whose body was as if it were made of rubber. No matter what shape he bent himself into, there did not seem to be any resistance whatsoever. He imparted an important message to the straggle of foreign travelers he had amassed around him: "Pity me," he'd cry out to them as they watched in awe, "I have to invent ever new ways to conjure up some form of sensation that will help me control my mind!" I also recall David Swenson saying that if your only objective was to master all six Ashtanga Vinyasa sequences, then you'd be at a loss once you'd achieved it. In truth, the objective is really always the same; simple in concept and yet so difficult in deed: to be totally present, in a nondual state of yoga or union. Even just to be in this state for one moment in an entire sequence is a great achievement indeed!

Different teachers have found varying ways to express this idea. Iyengar once famously stated, "alignment is enlightenment." When every single cell of your body serves the asana you are in, you do indeed become the embodiment of yoga or union. Edward Clark calls it "coalescence." The body moves into the most incredible positions with grace and ease. This does not mean it's "easy," because it requires unbroken concentration and great discipline. Until one has acquired the skill to consciously connect in this way, it is often much easier to surrender to habit and muscle through one's practice, than to flow with breath and gravity and really exploit the laws of physics in an intelligent way. But I promise you, it is worth it!

It is that rare and precious moment when you have positioned yourself in such a way, physically, pranically, and mentally, that you become the asana. The doer dissolves in the act of doing. It is the nondual state the sages have spoken about since the time of the Upanishads. It is that point of enlightenment when all is One and the mind is totally still. *Yogash Chitta Vrtti Nirodha* (Yoga is the cessation of fluctuations in consciousness). Clive Sheridan therefore vehemently urges his students to "pay attention!" These moments happen all the time, but they pass by unnoticed. Every time expectation meets fulfillment there is that spark of pure bliss, but as soon as the ego-mind gets in the way, it's over. So when your nose reaches that rose and it imparts its delicate fragrance, for just one moment there is peace. Immediately the thoughts rush in and the mind begins to label, categorize, judge, and analyze. Yoga teaches us to consciously cultivate that moment and to realize that you could be in it all the time, as it is nothing but a state beyond mind.

BEAUTY AND TRUTH: "THE GOLDEN SECTION"

Philosophers, mathematicians, and artists have been fascinated by the so-called golden ratio: when the sum of two parts and the larger part is in the same ratio as the larger part is to the smaller part. The ratio, which is approximately 1.618, appeals to the human sense of beauty and balance, and provides a mathematical constant, expressed in the Greek letter *phi*. Many yoga asana too reflect this sacred geometry, as can be seen in the image below. Philosophers such as Aristotle also spoke of the "golden mean" to denote a balance between two extremes, that of excess and the other of deficiency. This echoes Patajali's advice on balancing

sthira (effort) with *sukha* (pleasure) in all asana. The link between the aesthetic appreciation of beauty and the truths that pertain to human existence has been explored since ancient times in both East and West, and given its practical application in Quantum Yoga. The sublime nature of reality finds expression on all levels and in all modalities. It is up to us to refine our way of life in order to resonate with it.

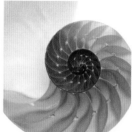

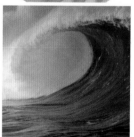

$a + b$ is to b as b is to a (1.618)

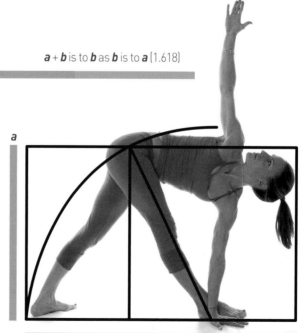

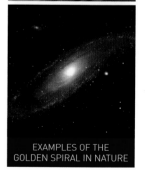

EXAMPLES OF THE
GOLDEN SPIRAL IN NATURE

THE TEN GROUPS

The ten groupings below sum up the musical symphony of
a Quantum Yoga sequence. It starts with a slow introduction
(Sublimatio); quickly gains tempo in Dynamic Flow (which
often consists of Sun Salutations; alternatives to avoid
straining the wrists or shoulders include squatting, horse-
riding stance, and *vajra-vinyasa* sequences); then once heat
and breath are established, a set of standing poses ensure
strong legwork, standing balances challenge focus and weight
distribution, and often dynamic inversions such as handstand
and forearm balance are practiced at this point. From here we
move on to a floor sequence, which typically peaks in one or
two particularly challenging postures, chosen in accordance
with the level of experience and the degree of challenge
appropriate on that day. Make sure to include forward- and
backbends, twists, hip-openers, arm balances, and core
abdominal exercises. Remember that the more complex asana
in particular can be a combination of these. We then move on
to the longer-held inversions (not for moon-day girls).

After a dynamic evening asana practice, definitely make sure
to include a shoulderstand to ensure that the vibrant energy
that has been generated through the practice is "earthed" and
the system calmed. Remember to elevate the shoulders off
the floor using neatly stacked blankets or four foam blocks
for anyone with a fragile neck. A morning practice can just
finish in headstand, although again if it was a very stimulating
practice it may be best to include shoulderstand also. The
counterpose to shoulderstand is *Matsyasana* (the Fish Pose),
but it does not always have to be done, as it is sometimes
very effective to roll out straight into *Savasana* (Corpse
Pose) in order to maximize the calming effect of the final
relaxation. A long-held *Shirsasana* (headstand) should always
be followed by the Child's Pose (*Balasana*) in order to avoid
the risk of stroke and release tension that may have built up
in neck and shoulders for those not yet so confident in the
pose. Remember that when practicing against the wall, the
interlocked fingers as in the classic headstand should be right
by the wall.

01) SUBLIMATIO
02) DYNAMIC FLOW
03) STANDING POSES
04) STANDING AND ARM BALANCES
05) FLOOR WORK: FORWARD-BENDS, TWISTS,
      SHOULDER AND HIP-OPENERS
06) ABDOMINALS
07) BACKBENDS
08) INVERSIONS
09) RELAXATION
10) MEDITATION

Below are indications of the percentages of time that should be allocated to the various groupings in accordance with the *dosha* one has set out to regulate.

QUANTUM SEQUENCE GROUPING PERCENTAGES PER DOSHA			
	VATA	PITTA	KAPHA
SUBLIMATIO	5%	8%	10%
DYNAMIC FLOW	15%	8%	20%
STANDING POSES	17%	10%	10%
STANDING AND ARM BALANCES	10%	8%	8%
FLOOR WORK	15%	13%	10%
ABDOMINALS	5%	3%	7%
BACKBENDS	5%	10%	15%
INVERSIONS	10%	15%	10%
RELAXATION	8%	10%	5%
MEDITATION	10%	15%	5%

01) SUBLIMATIO

DEFINITION

Sublimatio is the part of your practice in which you gently feel your way into your body and listen for the impulses that indicate both an intuitive and intelligent path to self-healing, spiritual growth, and a general improvement to the quality of your life. Here you turn the attention away from the involvement with the outer world towards a gentle interaction with the microcosm of the body-mind. The mind comes to rest in the immediate experience of your physicality, lovingly acknowledging how you feel right at that moment. You invite your thoughts to slow down, allowing you to be in the moment. Rather than look for solutions, you put your faith in the yoga practice that is about to unfold. You become conscious of the breath and slowly begin to introduce movement into the parts of the body that typically hold tension or stress. Before you introduce any weight bearing or impact to your practice, awaken the spine and loosen the joints to free energetic pathways.

Carl Jung borrowed the term *sublimatio* from alchemy, where it denotes a process of transformation from gross matter to gold. In psychoanalysis it means that negative emotions such as worry, anxiety, and limiting self-judgment are transformed into *rubedo*, reddening or warm feelings. The French philosopher La Salle explains: "Sublimatio is an ascent that raises us above the confining entanglements of immediate earthly existence and its concrete personal particulars." [12]

LISTENING

Sublimatio also refers to "inviting awareness," or "fine-tuning". What we are aiming for through Quantum Yoga practice is a state of awareness in every single cell of the body. Ultimately, we are practicing on the microcosm of our bodies a state of cosmic consciousness that extends beyond the confines of time and space. I have yet to meet somebody who is in a state of absolute mindfulness all the time. This does not mean it is inaccessible. "The cell is the bridge between the quantum world of unlimited possibilities and what we experience as reality." [13] Therefore, when you begin your practice, you must give yourself the time to listen and gently prepare for the process of transformation you are about to set into motion through your own will and effort. Remember that even the most exalted intention, without having first paid attention, can have undesirable results.

Listening does not mean analyzing or judging. "Negative" feelings or sensations should not be simply pushed or argued away, but lovingly acknowledged and worked with. In our practice we will often have to patiently address the physical results of incorrect movement, and identify the emotional charge that is at the root of these. We set out to reverse the downward flow of energy by harnessing the motivational force behind all these manifestations, and skillfully channel it through yoga practice. Remember, energy is energy. What you

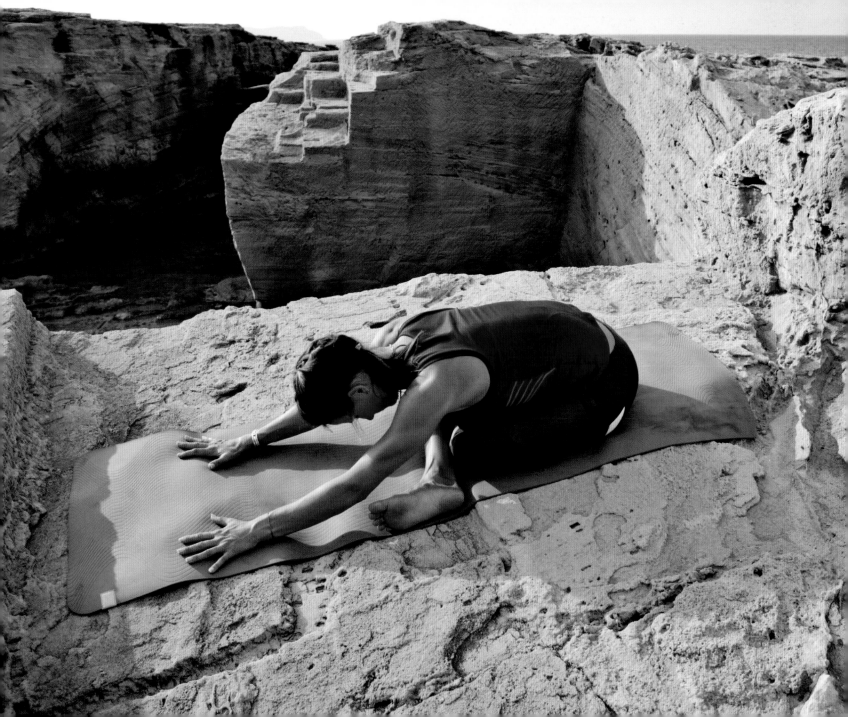

do with it is up to you. The passion behind the feelings that drag you down can be equally used to push you up.

The Buddhist concept of voidness, sunyata, describes the essential quality of all things as "empty." For instance, a sensation in your body is just that sensation, void of an inherent charge. Whether you label it as "good" or "bad," and therefore react with desire or aversion, is what affords it its qualities. Once you become conscious of this process, the way you respond becomes your choice. Herein lays your ultimate freedom.

Interestingly, quantum physics has now proven that anything pertaining to the material world really is empty in the literal sense. Matter consists of spaces. Once you look closer at the developments in science in the recent years, matter begins to seem a lot less tangible and real than energy. So if energy constitutes the charge that you give a thing, the reaction that your perception of that thing conjures in you, then indeed the sunyata concept is right. We think that an object's qualities are inherent, when actually it is we who give a thing its qualities. Under normal circumstances it is the ego-mind, which is shaped by our past, that determines how we react to things. Our field of experience is trapped in this binary world of desire versus aversion. We judge things by whether or not they are useful and right. This is perfectly appropriate for

operating in this world. However, the great mistake is that we believe that things are "inherently" such as we perceive them and that we have very little choice in the matter. Thus the quality of our lives is determined by circumstances. The truth, however, is that we have total control over our experience of reality and that things are as we chose to perceive them.

As yogis, starting with the sensations in the body and becoming aware of the reactions most clearly communicated by the quality of our breath, we seek to emancipate ourselves from this identification with what are essentially chemical reactions in the body. We can widen our scope of experience just by being with what there is, rather than reacting to what we think there is in a conditioned way. In the next step, through Dynamic Flow, we begin to actively cultivate equanimity through *vinyasa*, breath-synchronized movement.

IDENTIFICATION OF DOSHA

At this point, you will soon recognize the usefulness and application of Ayurveda in your choice or creation of yoga sequence. Can you identify any doshic imbalance? Put in simple terms, are you feeling and acting spacey (*vata*), fiery (*pitta*), or heavy (*kapha*)? How would you like to be? What mindset and energy level would be useful to you now? Fitness, weight loss, and greater inner calm are not the only benefits of yoga, nor are they limited to the time you practice or directly afterwards. More important are the deeper developments that affect the way you live your life.

If you are anyway fiery by nature, you will find temporary relief in the coolness you feel after you've sweated it out on the mat. But have you really worked on the fundamentals of why you are conditioned to push so hard? As for the health benefits, though you may feel satisfied by the reassuring ache in your muscles, how long can you sustain the calm before your organs are once again subject to the stress you create in your life, which weakens them?

If you are feeling heavy, stagnant, and uninspired, a gentle, meditative practice may make you feel temporarily light and lucid. But how long until you feel unattractive and depressed again? This is the time to stop analyzing and just get things moving through a more dynamic practice.

You may feel a little unsettled and anxious. A flowing, free practice will make you feel connected and cosmic, but for how long? Strengthening, grounding, and connecting with Mother Earth is what you actually need, because only if you're rooted can you play with confidence and be constructive in the process.

CHOICE OF THEME, PEAK AND SOUND

You may, at this point, want to choose a theme for your practice and perhaps even identify a peak pose or poses you'd like to work towards. Remember that there are often days that you may not feel in the right mind-set to create anything new, in which case choose from one of the Quantum Sequences and work on that! Also, if you would like to stray a bit, be a rebel and mix and match the different groups but adhere to the sequencing laws. Unusual variations often spontaneously reveal themselves to your consciousness as you go along.

As Sublimatio is about listening, this is also a good time to use sound to awaken our awareness of more subtle vibrations. If you have the luxury to practice in nature, ask yourself, what can I hear and how does it resonate with my inner nature? Otherwise you could also make your own sounds or chant mantras. Finally, you could consider what kind of music would be appropriate to support your practice or whether it would be more beneficial to just listen to your breath.

CENTRAL AIM

As explained in Chapter 2, the primary aim of Hatha Yoga, an umbrella term denoting the physical practice of yoga, is to bring prana into *sushumna nadi*. Combining *pranayama*, *bandha*, and asana, the flow of the *vayus* (winds) is manipulated in such a way as to ultimately strengthen the upward flow of prana *vayu*, encouraging the latent reservoir of energy (kundalini shakti) that lies dormant near *muladhara* (root) chakra to rise. This energy is accumulated at *ajna* chakra (eyebrow center), where it triggers an expansion and ultimately a permanently altered state of consciousness. This process involves and affects the gross and subtle bodies and therefore will manifest in physical, psychological, and mental transformation. Although the ultimate rising of kundalini is a mystical event, characterized by an extended period of trance, every yoga practice that is carried out in a selfless attitude, with skill and awareness, will enlighten the practitioner, making one energetically lighter and brighter.

SPINE

Sublimatio thus begins by gently awakening the spine and conscious breathing into otherwise "obscure" parts of the body, such as the back and sides. *Sushumna* (ray of light) *nadi* (river) is the central flow of energy in the body and runs along the spine. Therefore, your initial exploration of the body should start with the spine. Such gentle "Awakening the Spine" exercises can be done lying on the back or on all fours, such as in the Cat Pose. Can you identify parts of the spine that feel particularly tight and others that are very mobile? As the spine consists of sections that all affect each other, such imbalances are often mutually caused. So, if one part

is hypermobile, it is not allowing the stiff parts their natural range of movement, and conversely, the reluctance of the stiff parts forces unnatural mobility in others. Right at the start, you should aim to get the spine moving in balanced harmony and the rest of the body will follow suit.

JOINTS

Joints are the most vulnerable parts of the body, as with any machine, this is where one part connects to the other. Therefore, any weight-bearing exercises or impact through jumping and other dynamic movements should be preceded by a gentle opening of the joints to their full range of movement. Joints are slowly brought into motion through circling movements in both directions. These often generate clicking noises, which are nothing to be alarmed about. Yet, I would take note if there is a particular joint that clicks abnormally often and loud, as this is invariably a way of your body telling you that you are overstraining the joint or holding it locked in an unnatural position.

KEY AREAS OF TENSION OR INJURY

In Sublimatio, the practitioner should address the areas where they tend to hold tension. For most people, these are located in the shoulders, neck and jaw, the hips, knees, and often the feet as well. Problems are usually a result of an overreliance on furniture, strain through repetitive movement, the constant wearing of inappropriate shoes, and exposure to stress in general. Of course we do hold our emotions in our body and often even ancient karmic residue is said to lie at the root of dis-ease, but this should not stop us from recognizing simple lifestyle shifts that could alleviate much of the pain.

It is also in the Sublimatio section, right at the start of your practice that you should carry out any restorative exercises that may have been given to you by your physiotherapist or osteopath after an injury. Should there simply be particular parts of the body you feel you need to strengthen or ease up, focused work on these areas can also be woven in at a later stage.

MARMA OR AYURVEDIC PRESSURE POINTS AND SELF-MASSAGE

Most asana are designed in such a way as to stimulate the body through key pressure points in the body, referred to as *marma*, or energy junctions, in Ayurveda. One very powerful point I often use in Sublimatio is the eyebrow center, placing the hands in *anjali* mudra (prayer) with the knuckles of the thumbs between the brows. This gentle pressure supports the turning inward of the gaze.

When I have pain in certain joints or just feel particularly stiff, I like to give myself a brief massage in these areas, while sending them loving healing. I often use natural balms

that are mildly anti-inflammatory and decongestant or have an otherwise desired aromatherapeutic effect.

BANDHAS AND BREATH CONTROL THROUGH UJAII PRANAYAMA

Mula Bandha is one of the aspects of Hatha Yoga practice that is most misunderstood. It is primarily a psychic lock, meaning that the awareness and intention that lies at the root of it is far more important than its physical manifestation. Nevertheless, the root lock consists of a gentle contraction at the perineum, which is the muscle that lies between the anus and genitals, and a pulling up of the pelvic floor. Unfortunately, what often happens is that the practitioner ends up tightening the entire area, causing undue tension. Hence the exercises given in the Sublimatio section of the "Lotus Mandala", which lead towards a recognition of and control over the different sets of muscles at work here. It may be helpful to visualize the muscular set-up here as an eight-shape; the *mula* lies where the lines cross. This is not an area people tend to talk about freely, but let it be known that the majority of people experience some level of incontinence with age. This can be avoided through yoga.

Mula bandha represents the beginning of the ascent of energy, instigated from our root. It is the pulling up of our attention, away from our base concerns with survival that are rooted in fear, towards a higher intention. From the very root of our

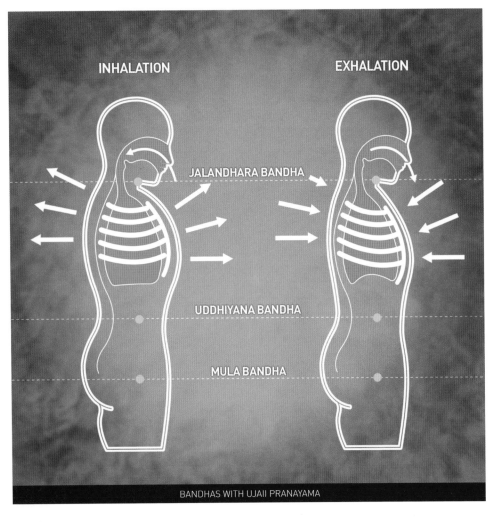

INHALATION

EXHALATION

JALANDHARA BANDHA

UDDHIYANA BANDHA

MULA BANDHA

BANDHAS WITH UJAII PRANAYAMA

body we are directing our efforts towards the cultivation of an enlightened state of consciousness. The things that drag us down do so because we allow them to. This may sound harsh and oversimplified, but the truth is that we have a choice in how we process the events of our lives. With disciplined and regular application of *mula bandha*, and the physical and psychological lift that it brings, you are snapping any self-denying tendencies at their root.

Uddhiyana Bandha, the abdominal lock, is the drawing back and up of the navel towards the spine and the dropping of the tailbone. *Uddhiyana* literally means "flying up"—it connects with *mula* to ensure an upward flow of energy. Once these two *bandhas* are engaged, one will often notice a subtle shift in weight distribution towards the heels of the feet. Most of us tend to unduly lean forward, as this is the direction in which we move and the location of our dominant sense of sight. Our stance will now support an awareness of where we are, rather than being always so concerned with where we are going.

It is a common misconception to think that yoga practice is all about flexibility, as it is as much about strength—specifically the strength to establish and sustain a posture and inner engagement that supports a balanced energy flow. Correct application of *mula* and *uddhiyana bandha* should ensure pelvic stability, which is often particularly hard for those who are naturally flexible. Furthermore, although the spine is beautifully designed in a double s-curve that ensures the greatest shock-absorption (SEE ILL.2), in many people this s-shape is exaggerated, particularly in the lumbar region. The aesthetic problem most people have with this is that the belly flops forward and the bum sticks out. From a health concern, insufficient core strength commonly results in back pain. Also, it is not healthy for the organs to be permanently distended. *Uddhiyana bandha* massages and tones the organs, and this effect can be increased with *nauli*, explained below. Certain styles of yoga and Pilates tend to overemphasize this point. Instructions like "*Mula bandha*, tuck it under!" are not helpful, as these more often than not result in a pushing forward of the pelvis and an unnatural loss of lumbar lordosis.[14]

Jalandhara Bandha, or the chin lock, is a drawing back of the chin, as if to form a slight double-chin. The result of a correct application of *jalandhara bandha* is that the neck feels like an integral part of the spine, the shoulders release, and the upper back broadens. It also supports a more inward attention and a humble attitude of conscious receptivity. Finally, *jalandhara bandha* is essential for *pranyama* breath control.

The even application of these three *bandhas* ensures balance, as *mula* and *jalandhara* stimulate the parasympathetic

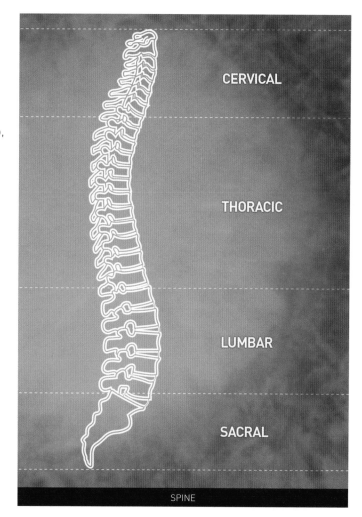

CERVICAL

THORACIC

LUMBAR

SACRAL

SPINE

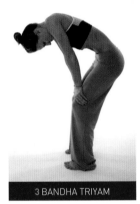

3 BANDHA TRIYAM

nervous system, and *uddhiyana* the sympathetic nervous system. These inner muscular grips or holds are referred to as "locks," as they lock the prana into the body. Furthermore, they manipulate prana in such a way that the upward flow is strengthened, giving the body lightness and grace and paving the way for the opening of higher consciousness.

The simplest way to strengthen this inner musculature and bring awareness into these parts is through *bandha triyam* (gripping of the three locks simultaneously) on *bhaya kumbhaka* (exhalation retention or empty). This exercise can be done in almost any position, but is easiest standing with feet hip-width apart, knees slightly bent, back rounded, and hands resting on the upper thighs (SEE ILL.3). *Bandha triyam* can be preceded by Lion Breath, which is a strong exhalation through the mouth while sticking the tongue out, which aids to clear the throat and release psychic waste. Also, the tongue is energetically linked to the root of the body and this exercise confirms this connection. All air is let out and then the bodily tissues are sucked back and up. I liken it to the effect of emptying the air out of a bag and then vacuum packing it. It is like a massive internal implosion back to one's core. The vigorous pulling back and up especially of the abdomen should be avoided by menstruating and of course pregnant women, as should the exercises described in the next paragraph. (See Chapter 5 for particulars.)

Two more practices that are categorized as *kriyas*, or cleansing exercises, can be done to great effect here, and are easiest first thing in the morning when the stomach is empty. *Agni sari* is a sort of fanning of one's internal flame. Yoga, and in particular this exercise, strengthens the *jiva agni* or "fire of life" that lies at one's core behind the navel area. This is why the body's ability to eliminate waste products is facilitated through regular practice. The healthy functioning of organs is supported and good metabolism ensured. One starts off again with a simple full exhalation, or Lion Breath, followed by *bhaya kumbhaka*, exhalation retention. Holding the breath out, one draws the navel back and up as before, but then repeatedly releases and pulls back up the abdominal muscles, thereby effecting a continuous backward and forward motion of the belly. Once this has been mastered, one should refine this movement by squeezing the central abdominal strands (rectus abdominis) together to then move only this in and out rapidly (SEE ILL.4). Remember to sustain *mula bandha* even as you manipulate the abdomen!

The next and far more difficult stage is *nauli*, or "churning" (SEE ILL.5 & 6), but like so many things that take patience and perseverance, it is well worth the effort. I always tell my students that if ever I gave up asana practice in favor of kite flying or scuba diving, I would always maintain the practice of *nauli*, as I believe it to be one of the most cleansing and strengthening practices a person can do.

Again, you start with the out-breath to empty, suck back and up, and then squeeze the central abdominal strands together, pushing them out. Then you direct them in a rotational movement. It is a veritable feeling of churning, as though someone had stuck a giant spoon into your *kumbha* (literally, "water pot" or "jar") and is stirring your inner soup. To start with just try to move the belly from side to side, and it is all right to hula-hoop the hips to encourage this motion. Make sure that you practice an even amount of times in each direction. Ultimately you will be able to keep completely still and rotate the abdomen rapidly one hundred times in one direction on a single *bhaya kumbhaka*, then the same in the opposite direction. I have heard different recommendations on which direction to go first, but as always I would recommend alternating. Most people find that moving clockwise is a lot easier than counterclockwise. This is because this follows the natural movement of matter in the body.

Here are a couple more pointers that may help you master *nauli*. You are releasing the spongy tissue of the organs back into the vacuum you've created through the exhalation retention, but conversely using the muscles to create the motion. So, the skill is to isolate the rectus abdominis but sustain the softness that is required for the rest to release back and up into the vacuum. Look at your belly while you do this. This will ensure *jalandhara bandha*, but also remember

that we are accustomed to our sight directing movement. Some of my teachers like to place the hands higher up than the thighs, right by the hipbones.

On a final note, do not get frustrated if nothing happens for a while. This is not exactly the kind of exercise you'd remember from PE class! Every time you concentrate on this area, you are building nerve passages that connect the conscious brain with these muscles. It takes a while to construct new roads, especially ones that run through resistant territories, where much physical and emotional debris is stuck, waiting to become unglued and finally be transported out.

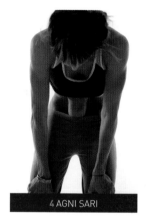
4 AGNI SARI

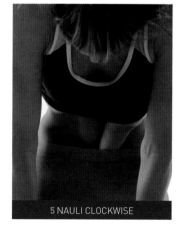
5 NAULI CLOCKWISE

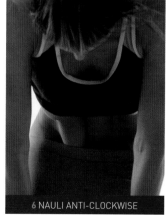
6 NAULI ANTI-CLOCKWISE

Having done these exercises, you have brought awareness into and strengthened the muscles in the key areas from which the harnessing and rise of prana is stimulated. You are not expected to hold these muscles in a state of hard and static contraction throughout your practice. Nor would this be conducive to anything but unnecessary tension. I recently went to a workshop held by two senior yoga teachers, during the Q&A session of which a disagreement between the two ensued. One argued that it was impossible to hold the *bandhas* throughout the practice while the other begged to disagree. In actual fact, they were simply talking about two different things. It is a common misunderstanding to think that *bandha* control means sustaining a permanent squeeze of the anal sphincter, pulling the belly in, and forcing the chin into the concavity of the throat. Ultimately, the use of *bandhas* was introduced in order to establish and promote the rise of *kundalini shakti* and the resulting expansion of consciousness. *Mula bandha* is your anchor point, the root of your intention to transcend the psychic blocks that are limiting you from self-realization. *Uddhiyana bandha* is your motor, with which you continuously support the "flying up" of prana. Any energy you accumulate is handed up with perseverance and skill, as it can easily get stuck at the seat of the ego near the solar plexus (*manipura*). Finally, *jalandhara bandha* ensures that during the time you have set aside for your practice, the precious pranic force you are harnessing is contained and not lost in interaction with the outside world through sense perception or improper breathing. What the *bandhas* lock you into is the state of yoga. They yoke you to your intention and cement your commitment.

Do not feel concerned if all this seems very abstract at first. Most people initially have no concept of what prana feels like. *Ujaii* breathing and the application of *bandhas* seem unnatural. Certainly sustaining them throughout the practice can strike one as totally impossible. Don't let this put you off! With time, through regular asana practice, you will develop this understanding and the control that comes with it, as these postures have been specifically designed to do. Therefore, begin with the most key pose: the Mountain.

TADASANA: THE MOUNTAIN POSE

Sublimatio gradually takes you up to standing. One should find time in Sublimatio to acknowledge that gravity does not equate with weight, but is a force that when consciously used can grant lift, especially when coupled with skillful alignment that respects the laws of physics and conscious breathing that exploits the upward pull of prana. As the body moves, one's center of gravity shifts. Coming to one's feet necessitates an acute awareness of the ideal positioning of the body with respect to one's center of gravity. This results in balance. If weight is evenly distributed, gravity pushes the body up.

The name *Tadasana* indicates that you should stand in such a way as to cultivate all the qualities associated with a mountain: powerful groundedness, integrity and heat at its core, and a cool, clear head like the lofty peak of a mountain. *Tadasana* is said to be present in each pose, when carried out correctly. In other words, one can find its essential qualities in each and every asana. It is a good idea here to work one's awareness from the foundation of the body up and visualize oneself as aligned along a central axis. The *meru danda* is the axis along which the entire world is aligned; and so the microcosm of your body should arrange itself along a *danda*, or medial line. As a yogi, you do this in such a way that reflects the natural order of things and unites you in harmony with the sublime flow of prana that permeates all beings with its divine essence. It is out of the endeavor to establish such an alignment that the *bandhas* should naturally grow.

Having established *bandha triyam*, *ujaii* or "victorious" breath should be introduced. *Ujaii* breath is the most misunderstood *pranayama* of all. Please take time to explore it either standing in *Tadasana* or even as a separate seated *pranayama*, before you move on to the Dynamic Flow, as it is much more difficult to sustain its even, steady, and smooth quality once you're moving. *Ujaii* is a method of breathing through the nose but with a gentle contraction at the back of the throat, which allows one to deepen, sharpen, and lengthen the breath

and thus bring it under control. It usually results in a gentle rasping sound that should accompany you throughout your practice. With the help of *uddhiyana bandha*, as you draw the breath deeply into the body, instead of the belly inflating, the ribcage expands in all directions. Prana is being pushed right down into the kidneys and contained with *mula bandha*. Through facia the diaphragm is attached to all parts of the body. Thus on the controlled out-breath, you will feel a natural release ripple through the body as the diaphragm lifts. The skill to synchronize this inner movement with the outer movement of the body is referred to as *vinyasa* and this is the central focus in the next section of the practice.

SUBLIMATIO POSES

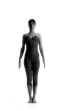 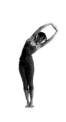 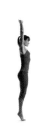 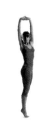

| TADASANA | TADASANA SIDE-BEND | VAJRA STANDING | VAJRA TWIST | VAJRASANA | VAJRA SQUAT & TWIST | FEET & SHIN STRECH |

| INTERLOCKED FINGERS | HOOKED THUMBS | | | WITH PROPS | | ROTATE JOINTS: HEAD, SHOULDERS, WRISTS AND ANKLES |

| BALASANA ARMS OVER | BALASANA ARMS OVER | CAT CONCAVE | CAT CONVEX | BADDHA KONASANA | LOW UTKATASANA | ROTATION IN PADMASANA |

ROTATE LIMBS IN A
CIRCULAR MOTION

| BANDHA TRIYAM | BANDHA TRIYAM | AWAKENING THE SPINE | JOINT ROTATION | SWASTIKASANA | PARYANKASANA | SUPTA VIRASANA |

| PADMASANA TWIST | PADMASANA SPHINX | PADMA SIMHASANA |

02) DYNAMIC FLOW

VINYASA

The primary objective of the Dynamic Flow section of the sequence is to establish *vinyasa*, or breath-synchronized movement. *Vinyasa* actually literally means "composition", but it is in such flowing compositions of movements that one can apply oneself to optimizing the interplay of prana and motion of the body in the field of gravity. If there is no time for a full Sublimatio, make sure at least to prepare with a standing *bandha triyam*. Thereafter spend a little time in *Tadasana*, Mountain Pose, running your mind's eye through the body from feet to crown, aligning and balancing yourself along your central axis and starting the conscious *ujaii* breath. Be attentive to the inner movement of the diaphragm that causes a very subtle sway. This *spanda*, or pulse, reflects the universal expansion and contraction. The skill to allow the internal movement of the breath to carry the external movement of the body will imbue the practice with lightness and grace. The effort to do so will ensure concentration and a refinement of the practice away from the use of brute force towards receptivity and flow. The resulting stream of consciousness can induce a trancelike state, but should not be mistaken for light-headedness. Again the fine balance between *sthira* and *sukha*, effort and receptivity, must be monitored constantly.

It is very important to understand that true *vinyasa* means allocating the same intensity and length of breath to each and every movement, no matter how difficult or easy it appears. This sameness in attitude and nondiscriminating mindfulness paves the way for equanimity. *Sam*, which denotes integration or wholeness, is the root of many spiritual concepts in Sanskrit, including of course samadhi, the eighth Limb of Yoga, and indicates that all aspects should be addressed with consistency.

With all yoga practice, we are learning to "get beyond the mind" and flow smoothly and in harmony with the supreme force. No longer do you want to get in the way of your self. Therefore, in the Dynamic Flow section, through repeated simple *vinyasa* compositions designed to allow the body to follow the lead of the breath, this attitude of receptivity is dynamically cultivated. You are consciously bypassing volition, so that it is no longer the ego-mind that decides, but the breath, which carries you. Allow for this deeply transformative process! Put all pushiness aside and instead patiently discipline yourself to initiate each movement with the breath. Breath takes the lead, the body-mind follows. With practice, this becomes automatic. You know when all parts "click into" this mode of being, because the feeling of freedom, strength, and grace is absolutely exhilarating.

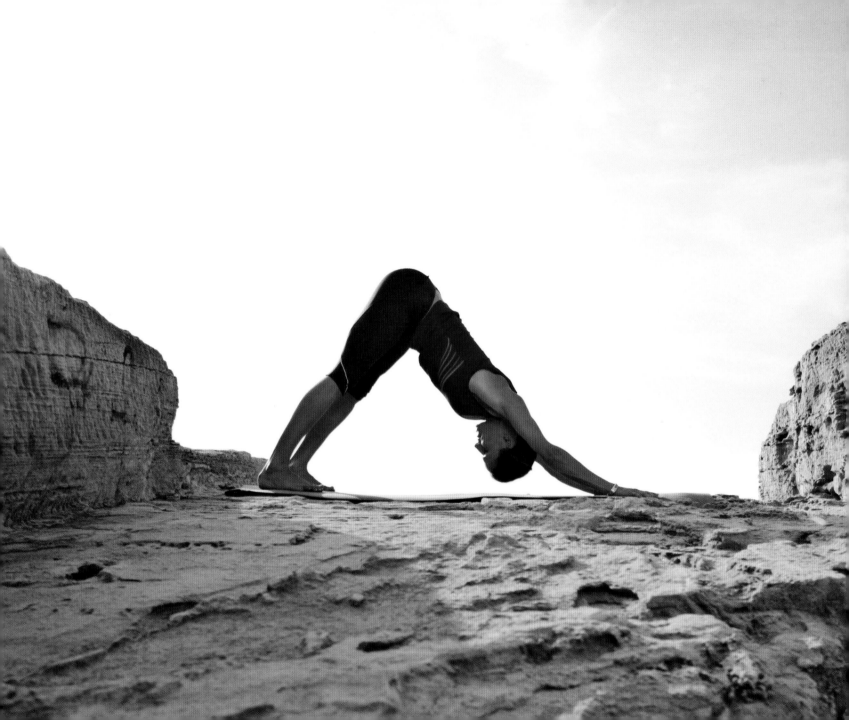

SURYANAMASKARA

Suryanamaskara, or Sun Salutations, make up a typical dynamic flow. Symbolically, these herald in the day and are done at sunrise. Some styles have also devised Moon Salutations (Chandranamaskara), which are said to be more suitable for sunset. However, it is ultimately your internal sun that you are saluting—the force within that gives life and throws light on that which was previously obscured. Yoga is about making the unconscious conscious. The expansion of space in the body leads to this widening of consciousness.

Traditionally, *Suryanamaskara* should be practiced daily without fail. The sun is the most powerful symbol of strength and perseverance. No matter what we humans get up to, waging wars on each other, exploiting the earth, and destroying nature in the process, the sun keeps rising every day. Such should be the consistent dedication of the yogi to the path.

Just as the sun takes its cyclical course, so you in *Suryanamaskara* should always come back to base: *Samasthiti*, standing upright and centered. When it is held, it is referred to as *Tadasana*, the Mountain Pose. *Samasthiti* means both "standing steady" and "all elements inert," referring to the stillness and sameness from whence movement and thus manifestation springs. It is also symbolic of the equality

and evenness with which the entirety of one's being is to be embraced in the practice of yoga.

I have listed a few *Suryanamaskara* options below, but there are of course endless variations. Again what is important is to sustain the rhythmic *vinyasa*! Where appropriate you can consolidate the postures within the composition with a full breath or more, but make sure to transit in and out on that side of the breath, which best serves the motion of the physical and energetic body.

ASHANGA A-TYPE
ASHTANGA B-TYPE WITH WARRIOR(S)
ASHTANGA C-TYPE WITH HANUMANASANA
SHIVANANDA SUN AND MOON SALUTATIONS
TRIPSICHORE BASIC SUN SALUTES[15]
BIRDS SUN SALUTATION INTO PIGEON AND LUNGE
LOTUS MANDALA SUN SALUTATION WITH FOREARM DOG & DOLPHIN

Note that in a *pitta*-regulating practice like the Heroes Sequence, the standing sequence is directly woven into the dynamic flow, in order to ensure even energetic expenditure. The Advanced Quantum Sequences[16] usually divide up into "sun ray clusters," in other words, Sun Salutation variations that weave standing poses, arm balances, floor work, and backbends into a varied flow

CASE STUDY: ADHO MUKHA SVANASANA

Let us here briefly discuss the Downward-Facing Dog Pose, or *Adho Mukha Svanasana*, as it is so widely practiced as part of the Suryanamaskara and *vinyasa*-links. Note that many of the points outlined in asana case studies here are universal and can be applied to other postures too!

As with any posture, we should build *Adho Mukha Svanasana* from its foundation upward. Unless one is deliberately working on a special effect, the hands should truly be in line with the shoulders and the feet as wide as the hips. Lining the joints of the individual extremities up in this manner allows for increased mobility. If, for example, the hands are too wide apart, the arms become like pokers that push the shoulders together. We discussed the three main *bandhas* at length in the last section, but there are many more. *Bandhas* denote areas of potential energetic leakage that results in a weakening of the entire structure. So a proper connection of the hands to the floor where they support the pose is referred to as *hasta bandha* (SEE ILL.7).

I'd like to point out here that since yoga means "union," the entirety of its practice deals with achieving (in Patanjali's Dvaita philosophy) or realizing (in Tantra and Advaita Vedanta) such a true connection. Ultimately, this yoga is between Atman, "the individual spirit," and Brahman, "the divine cosmic supersoul." So at any time that you connect two entities in a way that recognizes their essential oneness, you are practicing yoga.

Make sure that the middle finger is pointing forward, the hands are spread out, and the palms snuggled into the ground. The index finger knuckles and the thumb pads especially need to be held down. Keeping this firm connection to Mother Earth, one should endeavor to roll the shoulders away from the ears, shoulder blades gliding down the back toward the pelvis. The arms are straight. Beware, though, that if there is hyperextension in the elbow joint, it should be kept slightly bent to strengthen the muscles around it instead of taxing the joint. As for the feet, make sure that the heels are stacked right behind the toes, not collapsing in towards each other. Hit the roots of the thighs back and release from the knees down into the heels.

In the Downward-Facing Dog Pose, as with all other poses, bear in mind that the spine is the central focus, around which the body aligns itself. I am not a great fan of constant use of mirrors in yoga practice, as students should be encouraged to explore how the asana grows from the inside to serve their needs, rather than imposing an ideal outer form onto the body. Occasionally checking the outer form however can draw one's attention to areas that are being overworked and others that are left out. Also, as discussed earlier in the book, the use of simple geometric shapes to align the body will gradually bring it back to its true state of balance.

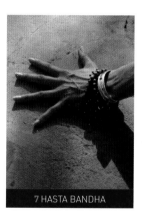

7 HASTA BANDHA

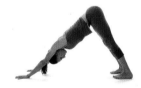

ADHO MUKHA SVANASANA

The Downward-Facing Dog Pose is an inverted-*V* shape, the apex being the tailbone. Check yourself out in the pose from the side, so you can see your profile in the mirror. The focus is on lengthening and strengthening the spine. Often in an attempt to get the heels to the floor, I see students scrunch up their spine, which defeats the general purpose of asana, namely to strengthen the flow of energy along the central channel. If this is the case, become longer in the pose! If, on the other hand, you feel that gravity is no longer supporting you in such a manner that you can lift your rear, but instead the extremities are sliding away from each other and the weight is collapsing forward, you have come too long, so you need to shorten.

The next thing to bear in mind is that the entire body should align itself along its central axis. The *bandhas* will support this, so that the belly does not flop down and the neck remains long. However, many practitioners give in to the temptation of collapsing the ribs down, so that the floating ribs poke out unnaturally. This gives you an obvious sensation of stretch, but contrary to popular belief, yoga is not simply about stretching. In fact, at many times, the informed and thus sophisticated practitioner will hold back on what I've come to call "sensationalism," that is, going for the obvious sensation. While the thoracic region goes into an exaggerated concavity as the ribs are pushed down, the lumbar is forced into a convex curve, causing in many bodies a visible bump.

The abdomen shortens and the shoulder blades pull together. The latter can be further aggravated if one strains to look at the navel. Though this is the official *drishti*, or viewpoint, of this pose, remember that *drishti* indicates in which direction the gaze should settle with a soft focus, so as to set a clear intention in the pose and support dharana, concentration. So if you still can't see your belly button even when the head is hanging down, the neck is relaxed, and the chin is gently drawn in, do not worry about it! You are looking in the right direction.

Another very useful thing to do in order to cultivate an even line of the spine in *Adho Mukha Svanasana* is to bend the knees. Throughout the basic Tripsichore Sun Salutes, the spine is worked in such a manner as to facilitate "the flow of energy along the *sushumna*," as Edward Clark emphasizes in his *vinyasa* teaching. To that end, the knees are deliberately bent in the Downward-Facing Dog in order to ensure the even line of the spine. However, if you do want to stick with the classical shape of *Adho Mukha Svanasana*, exhale and bring your knees to hover above the ground, inhale and arch the sitting bones up as high as you can (you can hold this for as many breaths as necessary, but again avoid pushing the ribs down), and exhale slowly while straightening the legs without losing the upward extension of the tailbone. If you're still in front of the mirror, see for yourself how this helps flatten a convex lumbar!

It may sound like a practical joke to beginners for whom this pose is everything but easy, but *Adho Mukha Svanasana* is classified as a resting pose. However, rest assured that what this indicates, apart from the fact that it does become easier relatively soon for most people, is that the energetic effect it is designed to achieve is stilling and balancing. You are gazing in towards the very center of your being. Behind the navel lies a point called the *kanda*, where all 72,000 *nadis* are said to cross and it is therefore the seat of power in the body. The arms and legs are worked in a very balanced way and the head is relaxed. One of my students once suggested that coming into Downward-Facing Dog is like coming home to an old friend. It is your harbor within the flow, where you can check your *bandhas* and alignment, emptying your thoughts into the even, steady *ujaii pranayama*, expanding into the infinity of the present moment.

CASE STUDY: CHATURANGA DANDASANA

When I teach the Birds sequence, I often liken the shoulder blades to wings, which can grant lightness, providing they are drawn down and wide, but placed *flat* against the back to support the opening of the lungs and heart region. Very often practitioners neglect these rules, which can cause damage if coupled with weight-bearing, such as in *Chaturanga Dandasana* (Four-Limbed Staff Pose), the Press-Up Position.

Chatwari, as the asana is often abbreviated, is not possible without proper application of *bandhas*, which ensures that the entire body hugs into its midline as though it were a staff, which affords lightness and supports the flow of prana along *sushumna nadi*. But there is more to it! The shoulders should be pulling back and away from the ears, the elbows should remain tucked into the torso so they are in line with the wrists and the neck is long. The chest is forward, open, and no lower than the pelvis. This allows one to smoothly proceed into *Urdhva Mukha Svanasana*, the Upward-Facing Dog pose.

Regretfully, more often than not, I see this asana done in such a way that the bum sticks up, the shoulders are hunched, the chest is restricted, and the elbows collapse out to the side, so that *hasta bandha* is lost and the wrists are strained. The transition into Upward-Facing Dog thus becomes a matter of force and the result is that the arch of the thorax is reduced and hence there is less space to breathe into. It comes as no surprise therefore that many yogis find it difficult to fully inhale at this point. All this could be avoided by keeping the chest somewhat higher in Chaturanga Dandasana whilst working the shoulders properly.

CHATURANGA DANDASANA

DYNAMIC SQUATS AND HORSE-RIDING STANCE VARIATIONS

This group of exercises represent dynamic flowing alternatives to the *Suryanamaskara*, and are usually variations on the horse-riding stance (*Ashvarohinasana*). These are particularly useful where wrist or shoulder problems do not allow the arms to bear any weight. Also, often one finds oneself without mat on a dirty or sandy surface, and in such a scenario these ensure that a *vinyasa* yoga practice is still possible. I have heard this group referred to as sthanas, but this is misleading as sthana means "the act of standing firmly'" "being fixed or 'stationary,'" or "position or posture of the body." You do of course want to cultivate a firm structure throughout, but at the same time flow with the breath.

Remember to start the practice with a simple horse-riding stance where the spine is neutral and the pelvis upright. In other words, you shouldn't stick your bum out and collapse the belly forward, nor overcompensate by thrusting the pubis unnaturally forward and tucking the tailbone under. (SEE ILL.8) It is useful to visualize the pelvis as a basin, which it is, filled with water. The water must not tip out the front or back. Also, pay attention to the feet. Imagine the feet have four corners. Distribute the weight evenly along these; in other words, don't let the knees collapse inward. From this pose, you can flow through the *Dhanushmat* (Archer) and *Lutasana* (Spider Pose) variations, or just do arm-strengthening exercises, visualizations, or chant the *bija* mantras, such as in the Heroes Sequence.

HEAT

The application of *bandhas* combined with the *ujaii* breathing is designed to strengthen the *jiva agni* or "fire of life," in the body, which is responsible for digestion and supports movement and elimination in the body. In *vinyasa*, dynamic movement is added to the equation and the resulting heat is intensely purifying and kick-starts the cleansing aspect of Quantum Yoga practice. Heat also softens the tissues and protects from injury. The use of heat to inspire and support the practice is inherent to the yoga philosophy. Even the ardent discipline and burning desire for self-realization which fuels the yogi's resolve is referred to as *tapas* (one of the *niyamas*, second Limb of Yoga). The root *tap* denotes heat. Therefore, even if you need to pause or rest at any time during the asana practice, keep the *ujaii pranayama* going! *Vinyasa* practice is about momentum, so don't stop if you get tired, but rather go slower and don't push yourself so far into the poses. Also, you could sneak in extra full breaths in the difficult transitions, but still remember to initiate each movement with the correct supportive breath.

BREATH AND MOVEMENT

As you become more confident and aware through Quantum Yoga practice, you will soon come to recognize the natural movement that the breath initiates. An inhalation is expansive and gives the body lift. The pelvis moves forward and the shoulders pull down. Unless it requires strength to lift the body off the ground, such as in *Urdhva Dhanurasana*, back-arches and bends are initiated with the in-breath, as well as any lifting of the arms and chest, and broadening of the sternum.

On the exhalation, the body pulls together and folds in on itself, which causes the pelvis to move back. Hence the feeling of release on the one hand, because of the drop in pressure, and power on the other, as muscles pull together. Therefore any movement that requires strength to bear weight or take an impact is usually initiated on the out-breath, as well as forward-bends and twists.

The next step is to exploit this subtle breath-body movement in such a manner that it takes you deeper into the asana. Here you are consciously imposing your will onto a natural motion, the awareness of which you have refined in this section through *vinyasa*, as you flowed with it dynamically. It is volition combined with skillful awareness of what is already happening.

Let's take the example of a standing back-arch, which forms the beginning of many types of *Suryanamaskara*. As you inhale, the arms rise and the body naturally arches; the out-breath would then take you into a forward-bend. However, if you decide to stay there and consciously set your will against the natural movement of the body, thus not allowing the pelvis

to move back and the stomach to pull together, but rather deliberately using the strength of the exhale to consolidate this expansion, the effect is that you move deeper into the posture. The torso lengthens and the feet dig more firmly into the ground. This process can be applied to all postures to great effect and its usefulness becomes most apparent in the more static sections that follow.

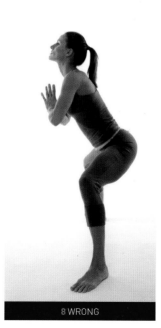
8 WRONG

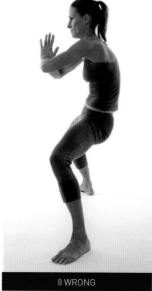
8 WRONG

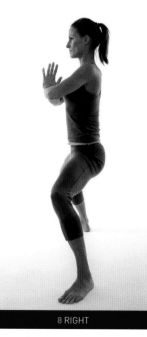
8 RIGHT

SURYANAMASKAR BASIC ASHTANGA STYLE

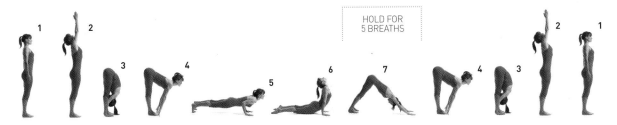

HOLD FOR
5 BREATHS

1 SAMASTITHI **2** URDHVA HASTASANA **3** UTTANASANA **4** ARDHA UTTANASANA **5** CHATURANGA DANDASANA **6** URDHVA MUKHA SVANASANA **7** ADHO MUKHA SVANASANA

SURYANAMASKAR WARRIORS ASHTANGA STYLE

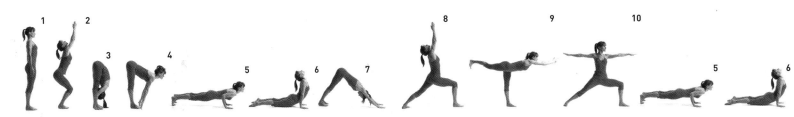

1 SAMASTITHI **2** UTKATASANA **3** UTTANASANA **4** ARDHA UTTANASANA **5** CHATURANGA DANDASANA **6** URDHVA MUKHA SVANASANA **7** ADHO MUKHA SVANASANA **8** WARRIOR 1 **9** WARRIOR 3

SURYANAMASKAR SHIVANANDA STYLE

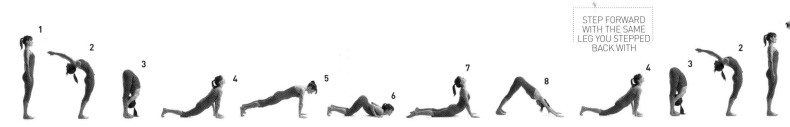

STEP FORWARD
WITH THE SAME
LEG YOU STEPPED
BACK WITH

1 SAMASTITHI **2** HIGH ARCH **3** UTTANASANA **4** LUNGE **5** PLANK **6** ASHTANGASANA **7** BHUJANGHASANA **8** ADHO MUKHA SVANASANA

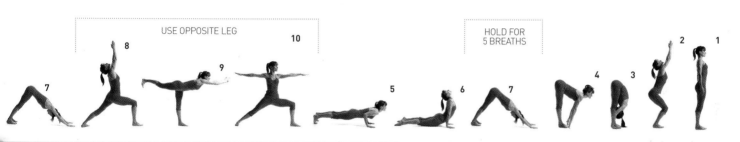

USE OPPOSITE LEG

10

HOLD FOR
5 BREATHS

7 8 9 10 5 6 7 4 3 2 1

10 WARRIOR 2

TRIPSICHORE BASIC SURYANAMASKAR

USE OTHER LEG

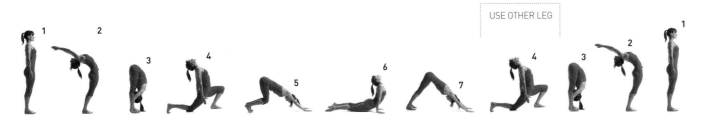

1 SAMASTITHI **2** HIGH ARCH **3** UTTANASANA **4** ANJANEYASANA **5** BENT-LEG DOG **6** URDHVA MUKHA SVANASANA **7** ADHO MUKHA SVANASANA

JOINT ROTATION & WALKING SPLITS SURYANAMASKAR

ARMS MOVE LIKE AN INVERSE BREAST-STROKE X 3

INITIATE WITH OPPOSITE LEG ON SECOND ROUND

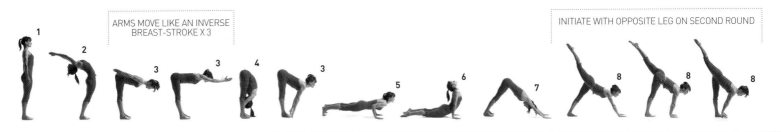

1 SAMASTITHI **2** HIGH ARCH **3** ARDHA UTTANASANA **4** UTTANASANA **5** CHATURANGA DANDASANA **6** URDHVA MUKHA SVANASANA **7** ADHO MUKHA SVANASANA **8** WALKING SPLITS

BIRDS SURYANAMASKAR

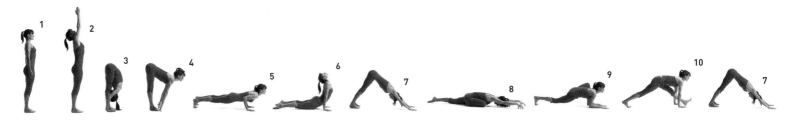

1 SAMASTITHI **2** URDHVA HASTASANA **3** UTTANASANA **4** ARDHA UTTANASANA **5** CHATURANGA DANDASANA **6** URDHVA MUKHA SVANASANA **7** ADHO MUKHA SVANASANA **8** EKA PADA KAPOTASANA

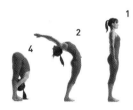

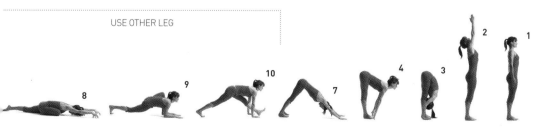

USE OTHER LEG

9 LIZARD **10** SPLITS PREPARATION

LOTUS MANDALA SURYANAMASKAR

USE OPPOSITE LEG

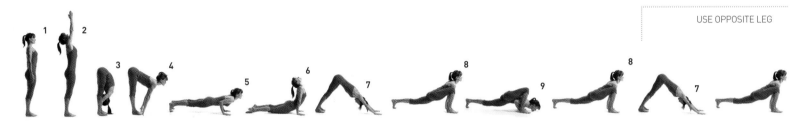

1 SAMASTITHI **2** URDHVA HASTASANA **3** UTTANASANA **4** ARDHA UTTANASANA **5** CHATURANGA DANDASANA **6** URDHVA MUKHA SVANASANA **7** ADHO MUKHA SVANASANA **8** LUNGE **9** LIZARD

DYNAMIC HORSE VARIATIONS

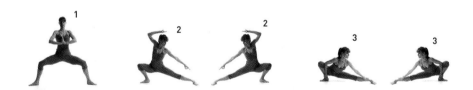

1 ASHVAROHINASANA (HORSE-RIDING STANCE) **2** DHANUSHMATASANA (ARCHER) **3** LUTASANA (SPIDER)

ASANA TO BE INSERTED INTO FLOW VARIATIONS

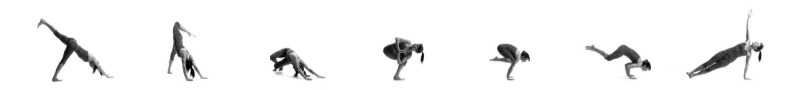

EKA PADA SVANASANA PARIVRITTA SVANASANA CROUCHING TWISTED DOG PARIVRITTA UTKATASANA BAKASANA CROW TO CHATWARI VASISHTASANA

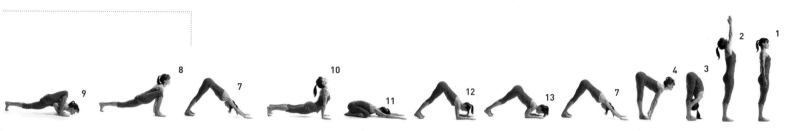

10 UP-DOG WITH TOES TUCKED UNDER **11** BALASANA **12** ELBOW DOG **13** DOLPHIN

VAJRA VINYASA

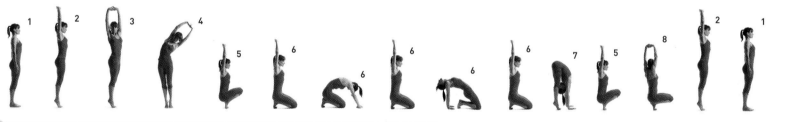

1 SAMASTITHI **2** STANDING ON TOES **3** TWISTING ON TOES **4** SIDE-BENDING ON TOES **5** VAJRASANA **6** VAJRA VARIATIONS **7** VAJRA UTTANASANA **8** VAJRASANA TWIST

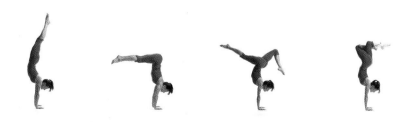

HANDSTAND   HANDSTAND TO CHATWARI   SCORPION-SPLITS STAND   EAGLE HANDSTAND

03) STANDING POSES

STANDING FIRM

The main objective of this section is to learn to stand firmly on your feet, no matter what is going on above. The human being is designed primarily to stand and move about on its feet. The way these connect to the ground in combination with the use of the legs determines the entire state of the body. Any posture, whether it is a standing pose or not, must be constructed from a firm foundation. If this is not the case, the rest of the structure will be shaky. If we establish strong leg and footwork first of all, then the rest of the practice will follow suit. The energetic effect of standing poses is primarily strengthening and grounding, even if a twist or side-bend is part of it. No matter what standing pose you are in, think about constructing it in such a manner that nobody and nothing could knock you over.

PADA BANDHA

We already discussed the ultimate standing pose, the Mountain or *Tadasana*, in the Sublimatio section, as well as the significance of *hasta bandha*, the hand lock, in *Adho Mukha Svanasana*. *Tadasana* is the simplest standing pose in which to explore *pada bandha*, the firm connection of the soles of feet to the ground. This level of connection should be sustained in each and every standing pose. Therefore place your feet at such an angle that allows for the weight to be evenly distributed on all four corners of the feet. Collapsed arches can be a real problem here. As they are a sign of an imbalance in *kapha*, lift is of utmost importance and is initiated through *mula bandha*, the root lock. Many traditions, such as Iyengar Yoga, lay great importance on the lifting of the kneecaps. Lifted kneecaps are an indication of good awareness in the legs. However, if you tend toward hyperextension, be particularly careful that you are really pulling the kneecaps *up*, rather than pushing the knees *back*. Locking joints often results in strain, weakening of ligaments, and slacking of muscles. Martial art traditions, where stability on the feet is crucial, expound that the energy flow gets blocked in locked joints. In my experience with yoga, positioning that is too static does not freely accommodate the divine pulse that beats at the heart of reality, to which as yogis we seek to be yoked.

FLAT- VERSUS SQUARE-HIPPED

Standing poses can be divided into two basic subdivisions: flat-hipped and square-hipped poses. Any midway point will not give you the full benefit of the pose. *Utthita Trikonasana* (SEE ILL.9), *Utthita Parsvakonasana*, *Virabhadrasana 2*, and *Prasarita Padottanasana* are flat-hipped. *Parivritta Trikonasana* (SEE ILL.10), *Parivritta Parsvakonasana*, *Virabhadrasana 1*, and *Parsvottanasana* are square-hipped. In the first group you are expanding within the invisible limits of a two-dimensional plane. In the latter, you are squaring the hips to the direction you are facing, and making sure as you move into the asana

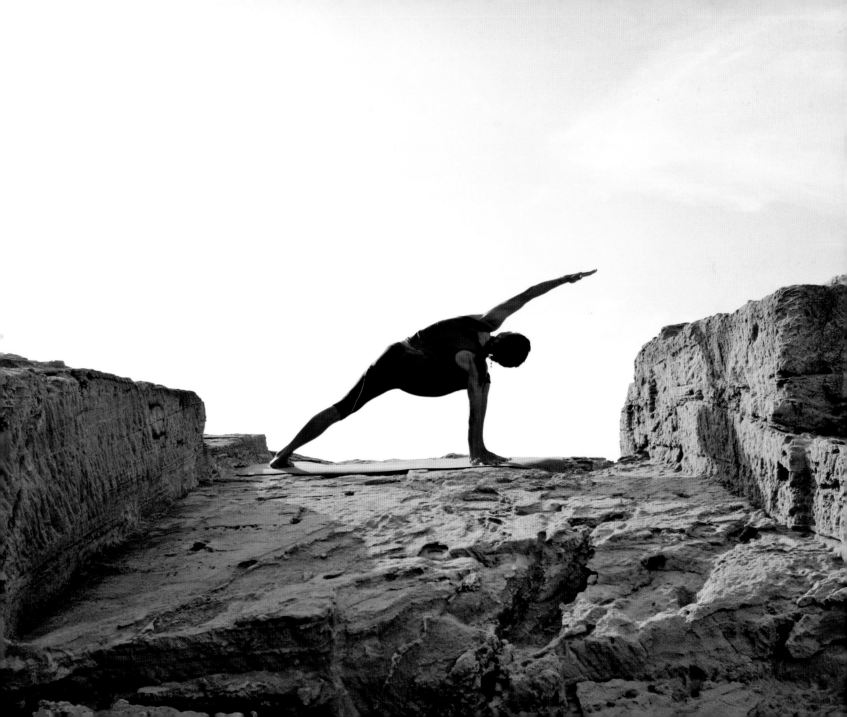

that the hips don't veer off to the side nor that one side collapses. In both cases, aim to remain centered along your medial axis. Alignment-focused schools, such as Iyengar, draw lines down the center of their yoga mats in order to encourage the students' awareness of this axis.

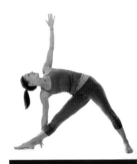

9 UTTHITA TRIKONASANA

ALIGNMENT

Quantum embraces the idea that perfect alignment in the domain of asana and beyond translates into clarity of intention. The general attitude and energetic focus must serve the pose, regardless of whether the outer physical body can actually yet achieve this form. Beginners often make the mistake of not setting their feet in accordance with the particular exigencies of each asana. In flat-hipped poses such as *Utthita Trikonasana* (Triangle), the feet are perpendicular to each other and in line. For square-hipped poses such as *Parivritta Trikonasana* (Rotated Triangle), the feet need to be positioned somewhat shorter and wider, and the back heel pulls back, so that the back foot is at a 45-degree angle. This allows the back leg hip to swing around and square up with the front leg hip. If you are wobbly on your feet, you will not be able to work deeply into the extension or twist of the torso. Therefore, first cut yourself some slack and become sufficiently familiar with the pose until you are stable. Then over time you can gradually come back onto the "tightrope" as flexibility increases and you gain steadiness on your feet.

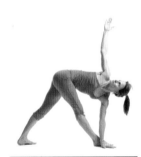

10 PARIVRITTA TRIKONASANA

GEOMETRY

Most standing poses are of a geometric shape. Why would we impose geometry on the organics of the body? There is a balance and perfection to geometric shapes that echoes the crystalline alignment we find when we study the subatomic level of the world and the macrocosmic level of the universe and planetary alignment. Yoga seeks to reconstruct this perfect state of balance within the physical and energetic body. Imbalances in our body are a result of behavioral patterns that reflect an internal psychological disturbance. The effect of submitting the body consciously to a geometric shape exposes these imbalances and thus brings them to our awareness. Remember the basic premise of yoga is to make the unconscious conscious. Acknowledgement paves the road for change. As we use these sacred asana to bring about a greater state of balance, the effect is threefold: Physically, the posture becomes more stable, and the improved structure allows the muscles to work more efficiently and the organs to function better. Psychologically, left and right brain use is balanced and we thereby tap into intuition with the backup of logic. Remember that when *ida* and *pingala* are perfectly balanced, prana gathers in *sushumna nadi*. Physical imbalances communicate a less-than-ideal flow of energy, and addressing these will in turn have a positive effect on vitality in general. Although the literal meaning of Hatha Yoga is under much debate by the academics, if we take it to mean harmony of sun and moon energy, male and female, heart and mind, the implication is that if we start by cultivating such balance in the gross physical structure of the body, a deeper internal balance will ultimately become established, too.

GRAVITY

Gravity is a force that is often mistaken with weight. As yogis, we learn to use this force in such a manner that it allows for a powerful grounding and yet at the same time gives us a natural uplift. It seems like a paradox, but the more you work with gravity, the lighter you become. So, this play with gravity outlines the ultimate challenge in your standing poses. How can you be both stable and light at the same time? How can your attitude be firm but relaxed? How can your relationship with Mother Earth be one of affirmation and yet nonattachment? By persistently challenging yourself to find this elusive state of balance in each and every asana, neither muscling through your practice nor slacking, you will stumble across solutions to life's greater questions when you least expect them. This is because the life–affirming attitude you are hereby cultivating leads to a state of sattvic (self-illuminating) clarity.

SPANDA

Many standing poses are designed with an upwardly or diagonally extended arm. We have spoken a lot about the central harnessing and manipulation of prana through the subtle contraction of the *bandhas*. This does not mean that we can forget the extremities. Just as we pull in, so we must also radiate out. The Anusara style of yoga places great emphasis on the idea of *spanda*, the universal pulse, in the context of asana. I will return to this concept later in the discussion of joints and binds, but here too it is useful. Often I see students who are grounded and strong, mostly the *kapha*-types, but whose stance is marked by a general heaviness, clearly revealed by a lazy top hand. The energy should radiate right into the fingertips of extended arms, and this in turn will give a lively dynamic even to static poses. The sense of sight communicates the direction of energy and thus the gaze should follow. *Jalandhara bandha* is very important in supporting *drishti*. When rotating the head to look up, make sure to draw the chin in, so that the neck remains an integral part of the spine. Sticking the chin out will not only create discomfort, but also put a kink in your pranic flow. In *Parsvakonasana* (see below) it is particularly difficult for the neck to harmonize with the spiraling spine, but it helps to look up from underneath your armpit, before directing the gaze past the outstretched fingertips. Draw the chin in as much as possible and exercise your eyes! Remember also that any stretch in yoga is an extension in *both* directions. Therefore, just as much as you are stretching into the fingertips, you are also pulling the shoulder away from the ear to make further space for the neck. Naturally this will make it more difficult to keep the elbow straight, but then nobody ever said that yoga is easy!

CASE STUDY:
PROTECTING JOINTS IN PARSVAKONASANA

Knees and wrists in particular are problem areas for many yogis. I discussed the warming up of joints through circular rotating motions in the Sublimatio section. Should you feel a strain at any point in your sequence, these motions can of course be repeated. Strain can be avoided through correct alignment.

Joints are at their most stable when they are stacked on top of each other. So, the bent knee in the *Virabhadrasana* (Warrior) and *Parsvakonasana* (Bent Angle Pose) variations should be placed above the heel and ankle, certainly not short of it. *Kona* means "corner" and what is meant is a truly right angle. The bent knee going beyond the ankle indicates a collapse of the pose, often accompanied by a loss of the back foot connection to the ground (*pada bandha*). Again remember that your priority is to be steady on your feet and that this will inform what goes on above.

So although the center of gravity is lowered through the bent leg in *Utthita Parsvakonasana*, the torso should be spiraling up and away from it, as you aim to bring your belly to face the sky. In this way it becomes a beautifully powerful, but dynamic pose.

Similarly, in the rotated version (*Parivritta Parsvakonasana*), one needs to sink into the legs, stabilize the back foot (even if you choose to lift the back heel up and tuck the toes under to stop the hip from veering out, you can stabilize by hitting

UTTHITA PARSVAKONASANA

the thigh back strongly and keeping the center of gravity low), and lift the chest to the sky. In the *Namaste* version, the prayer hands can facilitate the opening of the sternum. I recommend only going into the full *Parivritta Parsvakonasana* once you can stem your shoulder against the outer bent knee, without loss of the right angle, and thus involve the entire torso in the rotation.

PREPARATION FOR FLOOR WORK

The reason we place the standing poses before the floor work is mainly to protect the back. At this point the feet constitute your base forcing the legs into action. Later the foundation of the poses becomes bigger, so the legs tend to lose consciousness. Many back problems could be avoided if the legs remained engaged in the floor work!

SURVIVAL

Standing poses pertain to *muladhara* chakra. It is only once you stand firm and steady that you can overcome our natural preoccupation with survival. Your basic needs must be covered for any energetic assent to be successfully initiated. How could you overcome something that you have not yet mastered? How can you renounce something that you never had? Hence always include a few standing poses before you move on to more complicated and challenging postures.

HISTORY OF STANDING POSES

It is interesting here to note that neither the *Suryanamaskara* nor the Standing Poses are mentioned in the medieval scriptures such as the Hatha Yoga Pradipika, the Gheranda Samhita, or the Yogayajnavalkya. With *Suryanamaskara* it would be fair to say that knowledge of these may just have been taken for granted, so ancient are they said to be. Also, dynamic exercise may not have been as necessary, given the fact that most Hatha yogis were forest-dwelling ascetics, whose lifestyle demanded physical exertion. Asana practice however was primarily done in preparation for meditation, as well as for organic and energetic effect, so most asana we find here are floor poses such as hip-openers, twists, forward- and backbends and arm balances, as well as the inversions. *Asana* literally means "seat" and was primarily a way of building one's own throne to enlightenment.

Many yoga teachers nowadays justify the more standing- and movement-based practices they have developed by pointing to the traditional links between yoga, martial arts (in particular the Keralan Kalaripayat) and dance (Bharatnatyam from the South and Khatak from the North of India). I even remember one teacher claiming that he had gathered most of the information at his disposal from studying temple walls, while the rest was channeled directly from Krishnamacharya. This kind of self-authentication is the unfortunate result of the fact that historical proof pertaining to most things Indian is extremely difficult to procure. This vast and ancient culture began with the deliberately secretive Brahminical oral tradition (explained in Chapter 1), and much that was eventually written has meanwhile been lost or destroyed. Most importantly, there exists a pan-Asian reluctance to historical dating. This has a lot to do with the view of time as something cyclical rather than linear. Although this can be frustrating at times for historians and scholars, I personally find it an attractive worldview.

Some scholars argue that physical yoga as we practice it today was influenced by Western exercise ideals, gymnastics in particular. The introduction of British military drills and physical education—often in preparation for team sports—into Indian culture in the nineteenth century definitely had an effect. The cross-fertilization between Indian and Western culture may well be one of the reasons standing poses are so widely practiced today. The Triangle Pose may have been inspired by the jumping jack, and the Warrior Pose by the lunge. India has traditionally been tolerant of foreign cultures, while assimilating imported practices into something uniquely Indian. The Quantum Method embraces this natural development of yoga to cater to the exigencies of modern life, but encourages you to question which part of this life you chose, and which was imposed on you and could therefore be relinquished. With regular yoga practice, your body-mind will reveal this to you.

STANDING POSES

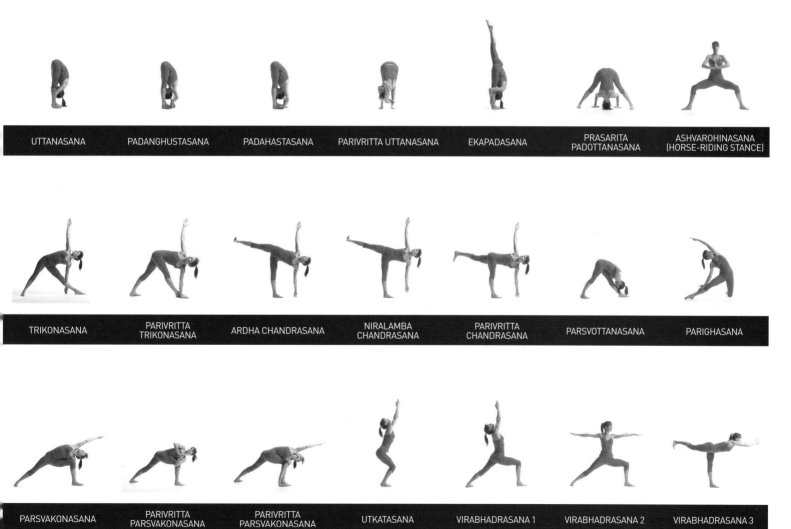

| UTTANASANA | PADANGHUSTASANA | PADAHASTASANA | PARIVRITTA UTTANASANA | EKAPADASANA | PRASARITA PADOTTANASANA | ASHVAROHINASANA (HORSE-RIDING STANCE) |

| TRIKONASANA | PARIVRITTA TRIKONASANA | ARDHA CHANDRASANA | NIRALAMBA CHANDRASANA | PARIVRITTA CHANDRASANA | PARSVOTTANASANA | PARIGHASANA |

| PARSVAKONASANA | PARIVRITTA PARSVAKONASANA | PARIVRITTA PARSVAKONASANA | UTKATASANA | VIRABHADRASANA 1 | VIRABHADRASANA 2 | VIRABHADRASANA 3 |

04) STANDING AND ARM BALANCES

DHARANA, DRISHTI AND BINDU

There is a direct link between balance and concentration. As previously discussed, the main reason for a lack of concentration (dharana) is the result of the senses' preoccupation with external objects. The mind represents the master sense and its preoccupation is with past and future, which lie outside the immediate experience of the moment. In order to focus the activity of the senses, we need to channel them into a single point. In vision this point is referred to as *drishti*. The higher the *drishti*, the harder the balance. The ultimate challenge is to rely on the inner *drishti*—closing the eyes in a standing balance and tuning into our internal capacity to stay aligned along our central axis. Once again the physical effort of the body to hug into its medial line results in an energetic pull towards the center, increasing the pranic potency of the *sushumna* (ray of light) that runs through our very being.

Good balance is never a result of rigidity. Quite to the contrary, it is a matter of yielding and yet remaining aware of one's center. In Asia, the bamboo is regarded as the strongest tree, because due to its capacity to yield to the wind, it is often the one that does not break in the storm. Similarly, any focus in yoga is a soft focus. One is not observing an object in the conventional sense, but rather looking through a single point into infinity. In essence a point is a nonentity anyway

and our vision thus dissolves into the eternal void. Even within the head, at about the height of the pineal gland, we carry the *bindu* or point of emanation as well as dissolution of the universe, so we all carry the very source of existence within. All dissolves into that point and yet it is from whence we emanate.

In standing balances we have further decreased the surface area of our foundation and destabilized the weight distribution. The challenge is the same as in the standing poses: to be grounded and yet lifting internally to make us lighter. The latter is even more important here. If you think about it, in order to fly, you need to increase your surface area versus your weight. So really in a standing balance you are expanding the breadth of your attention, while staying focused on one point. Even if you don't yet grasp the *bandhas*, you will be automatically internally pulling up and constructing the posture in such a manner that compensates for the redistribution of the force of gravity.

COUNTERBALANCE

Physics reflects the laws of nature in general. What you take away, you must give back! You should use opposing forces cleverly in order to strike a state of perfect balance. The Tree Pose (*Vrikshasana*) variations provide a good example: when you move into Side-Bending Tree (SEE ILL 11A), as you arch over

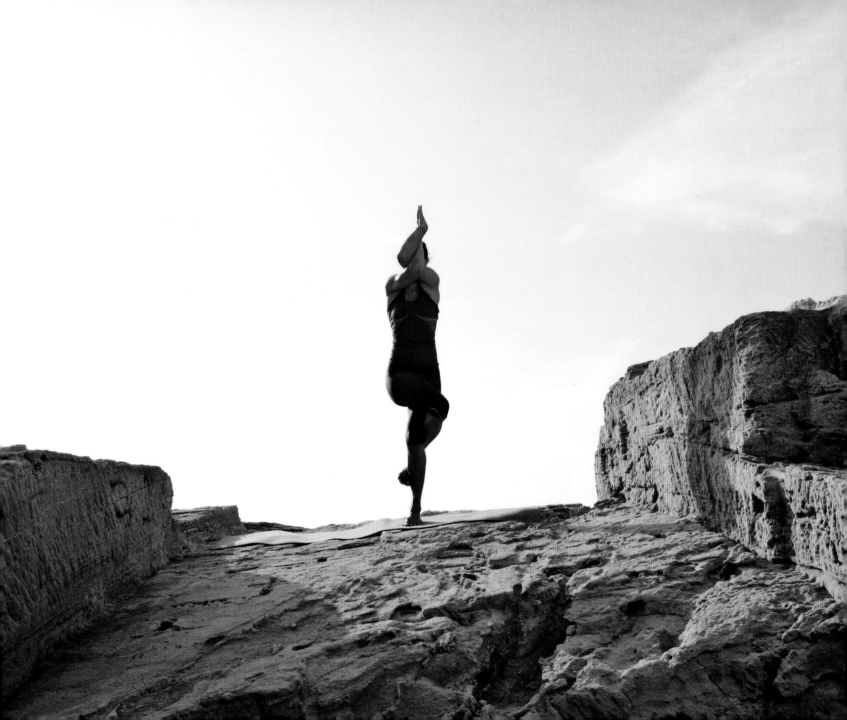

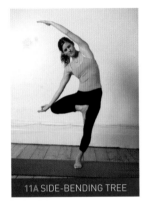

11A SIDE-BENDING TREE

to one side, at the same rate you need to push the hips to the opposing side. Similarly, when you go into Toppling Tree (SEE ILL.11B), in the same measure that you reach the outstretched limbs up to the sky, you should release the torso down. This needs to be done gradually, and the breath can help here. Inhale, stretch up; exhale, release down. With such subtlety you will eventually master all balances!

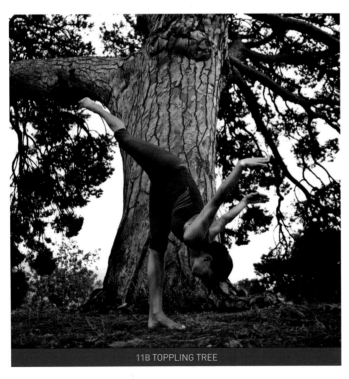

11B TOPPLING TREE

HANDSTANDS AND FOREARM BALANCES

Arm balances can also be brought into the sequence at this point, especially the energizing inversions Handstand (*Adho Mukha Vrikshasana* or Downward-Facing Tree Pose, SEE ILL.12) and Forearm Balance (*Pincha Mayurasana* or Peacock's Tail-Feather Pose, SEE ILL.13). In essence these are backbends, and herein lies the catch-22: in a sense, it is safer to practice freestanding handstands and forearm balances at the end of the backbending section, for if you fall, you should then easily drop into a backbend. However, if you want to learn to hold a free-standing balance in these inversions, you need to cultivate the upright, pole-like feeling of *Tadasana*. I often practice *bandha triyam* on *bhaya kumbhaka* (see *Sublimatio* section, Chapter 3) again here, in order to tighten the core, so as to avoid dropping over into *Urdhva Dhanurasana* (Upward Bow Pose). Energetically too, it makes sense to practice these again at the core of your sequence. The handstand and forearm balance are often regarded as advanced postures and indeed they seem scary and hard for the beginner. Although caution is of course advisable, certainly if you practice them against the wall and initially under the guidance of a qualified teacher, the poses in themselves contain nothing that is beyond the beginner's grasp.

There are many ways of coming up into a handstand. The most useful way to practice it in the beginning is with the bunny-hop, both legs working as a single unit. Try this at the wall first, the hands shoulder-width apart, about a hand-length from the wall. Really discipline yourself *not* to kick up with one leg. Also, those with open hips need to make a real effort to keep the legs *together*! A common mistake with the bunny-hop is that the heels are yanked up, which causes the lumbar region to collapse into a backbend. Think of your legs as the strong hind legs of a mighty hare, and push forward so that your sacrum moves in the direction of the wall. Do not straighten your legs until the soles of the feet are against the wall. The objective is to stack the pelvis over your shoulder-girdle *before* you straighten the legs. Also, with bent legs, part of you is still forward-bending (in gymnastics this is referred to as a *pike*). As you straighten the legs slowly and with control, be mindful to preserve the erectness of the spine with the help of *mula* and *uddhiyana bandha*.

Adho Mukha Vrikshasana means downward-facing tree. Use the wall to support that pole-like feeling, your inner *Tadasana* as it were. Push up strongly through the straight arms, reach the legs to the sky and do not lose the *ujaii* breathing or *uddhiyana bandha*. Eventually you should come off the wall as a result of this erectness, rather than ending up in the unfortunate position with the heels against the wall, the belly flopping forward, and the back jammed.

Another way of coming into handstand is from *Ekapadasana*, the Standing Splits. This pose is more useful for advanced practitioners, as it requires a certain amount of flexibility in the hamstrings and good breath and bandha control. On the inhalation the leg draws up, whilst the weight moves forward and into the hands. Then on the exhalation, the upwardly extended leg should literally pull the standing leg up to it. At the beginning you will be tempted to hop, but with disciplined practice, you will no longer need to. The same can also be done in the forearm balance. It is well worth overcoming the need to kick off, not merely because it is far more graceful and in harmony with the breath, plus bending the standing leg knee takes your centre of gravity down again, but also because kicking off is what usually makes one fall over.

Pincha Mayurasana literally means "Peacock's Tail-Feather Pose." As it has a bigger base and allows for more of a curve in the spine, the balance is easier to maintain. However, tightness in the shoulders and dorsal region can make it very difficult to come up in the first place. The objective is to align the hands, wrists, and elbows parallel to each other, shoulder-width apart. Forearm Dog and the Dolphin prepare directly for it. Here you will soon realize whether your elbows tend to slide apart, in which case the use of a brick and a belt can be very helpful. Place the wide side of the brick against the wall. Make a loop with the belt and place it just above the elbows; the size of the loop should ensure that the

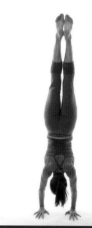

12 ADHO
MUKHA VRIKSHASANA

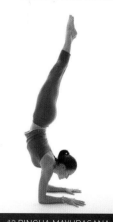

13 PINCHA MAYURASANA

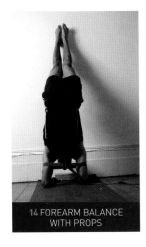

14 FOREARM BALANCE WITH PROPS

elbows remain shoulder-width. Wrap thumb and index finger around the edge of the brick and ensure good *hasta bandha*, pressing the index finger knuckles and thumb pads into the ground (SEE ILL.14). Your *drishti* is on the edge of the block between your thumb-tips. Now walk your sacrum as close to the wall as possible. Here you can kick up one leg at a time, but make sure to immediately pull the legs together with the help of mula bandha. Avoid collapsing the back by tightening *uddhiyana bandha*. Push the forearms firmly into the ground and breathe steadily. Be especially careful coming down from *Pincha Mayurasana*. As the legs have to circumscribe quite a big arch, the feet can come down with some force, so be mindful of your toes!

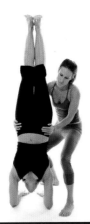

15 FOREARM BALANCE ADJUSTMENT

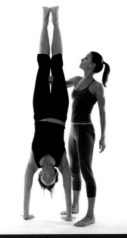

16 HANDSTAND ADJUSTMENT

If you have someone to initially help you up, make sure they keep their face out of the way. It is the practitioner's responsibility to pull the legs together as much as possible, but beware that even with the best of intentions, legs have a tendency to flail, especially when the person panics. The adjuster should know that the best place to hold a person is at the hipbones (SEE ILL.15), but again this may take some practice and getting used to. Particularly in handstands, it is surprisingly effective for the adjuster to place a clenched fist between the yogi's thighs, which the yogi then presses together strongly (SEE ILL.16). Often you will find it possible to balance with just that!

Please note: handstand drop backs, Scorpion (*Vrischikasana*) variations, and flicflacs do require the spine and shoulders to be prepared with backbends (See *Backbends* section, Chapter 3). Other variations such as those that involve going into Lotus should be placed within the Floor Work section, once the respective body parts have been opened up.

PROTECTING JOINTS: ARM BALANCES

When the arms bear the weight of the body, careful attention to joints becomes even more crucial than when on your legs. So, for example, in *Vasishtasana* (Side Plank Pose), try aligning wrist, elbow, and shoulder vertically above each other and you will immediately find that it feels like you are carrying less weight. Don't lift out of the shoulder joint, but release back into it.

In the *Bakasana*, or Crow Pose (SEE ILL.17) (and also in the Three-Point Headstand), make sure that the elbows remain above the wrists and don't collapse out to the side. If they do, chances are you are scrunching up your shoulders and working with brute strength. If they don't, you are allowing for lightness.

Another indicator of potential strain to wrists and ankles is the flesh around the joint. Be attentive to the creases around the joint. Are they even? If they are not, you may need to place your hands or feet at a different angle. Flesh that is unevenly scrunched up is a dead giveaway that you are not working in a balanced way. Your aim is to structure all asana in such a way that is in accord with the laws of physics, in keeping with the organics of the body, and allows a smooth pranic flow.

FLOWING IN STANDING POSES, BALANCES AND FLOOR WORK

At this point, I would like to encourage the Quantum yogi to consider how asana can be linked dynamically. When confronted with a posture that is new to you, first explore it as a separate entity. However, crossovers and curious ways of linking will soon reveal themselves to you. You will find many examples in the Quantum Sequences given. The more advanced the sequence, the more complicated these can be. To make your own, use a certain part of the posture as a leitmotif. This could be the Half-Lotus or Half-Pigeon leg; a

certain hand mudra; different variations of a squat; varying lengths and widths in the same pose; or doing a forward-, side-bend, and twist in the same pose. Start off slowly with these experimentations and be mindful to balance the two sides. Above all, have fun with it!

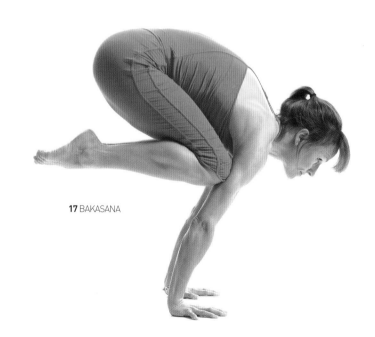

17 BAKASANA

STANDING AND ARM BALANCE POSES

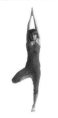 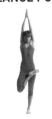 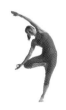 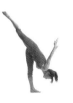 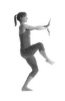

| VRIKSHASANA | PADMA VRIKSHASANA | SIDE-BENDING TREE | TOPPLING TREE | SHIVANATARAJASANA 1 | SHIVANATARAJASANA 2 | SHIVANATARAJASANA 3 |

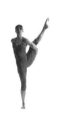 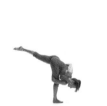 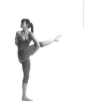

| BOUND PARSVAKONA BALANCE | BOUND PARIVRITTA PARSVAKONASANA BALANCE | BAKASANA | PADMA BAKASANA | TITIBHASANA | TITIBHASANA |

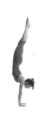

| ADHO MUKHA VRIKSHASANA | SCORPION-SPLITS | PINCHA MAYURASANA | UGLY ASANA |

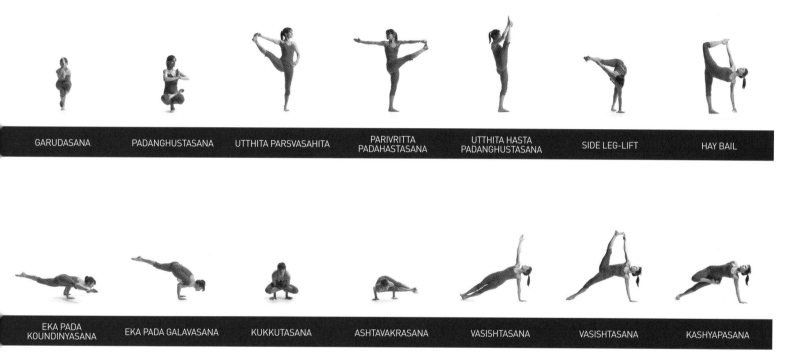

GARUDASANA   PADANGHUSTASANA   UTTHITA PARSVASAHITA   PARIVRITTA PADAHASTASANA   UTTHITA HASTA PADANGHUSTASANA   SIDE LEG-LIFT   HAY BAIL

EKA PADA KOUNDINYASANA   EKA PADA GALAVASANA   KUKKUTASANA   ASHTAVAKRASANA   VASISHTASANA   VASISHTASANA   KASHYAPASANA

05) FLOOR WORK

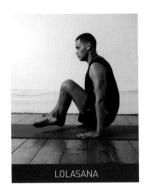

LOLASANA

The floor work section consists of forward-bends, twists, hip-openers and composite poses. The culmination into a peak pose, if one has been chosen, happens either here or after the backbending section. Let me remind you again to please not lose consciousness in the legs at this stage! It is in this section that the *sthira*, the steadiness in the practice, often falters, which is communicated through shallow, irregular breathing. A disregard for the stability of the base of the respective poses can be cause for injury and leave you with an ungrounded feeling.

In the event that you have deliberately chosen to do a more "yin" practice of receptivity and surrender, cultivate a total discipline of relaxation. (*Yin* is taken from the Chinese cosmology and denotes the feminine, as opposed to yang, masculine principle.) In other words, challenge yourself to keep every muscle and thought soft. You could even use a blindfold (a cotton or silk scarf tied around your head will suffice); temporarily impeding the sense of sight induces partial *pratyahara*, and the gentle pressure on the eye cavity brings further relaxation. Props can be very useful here, such as in a restorative practice in general. (See Chapter 5).

The use of so-called half and full *vinyasas* (for example, Chatwari, Upward-Facing Dog, Downward-Facing Dog, and Jump-Through) such as in Ashtanga Vinyasa may not

be particularly imaginative, but when done correctly can be effective and strengthening. Unfortunately more often than not, they are done incorrectly. By regularly practicing *Lolasana*, the Earring Pose, you will be prepared. Remember that the hands should be shoulder-width apart, beside the hips. As you lift yourself off, suck up using the *bandhas* and make your trunk into as compact a ball as you can. Then try to swing back and forth like a dangly earring. Eventually you should be able to ride the momentum and shoot your legs back into *Chaturanga Dandasana*, the Press-Up Position. It takes a while to learn this and can be very frustrating. My recommendation is to always initiate the *vinyasa* jump-through properly, in other words, with the hands beside your hips, lifting your body off the floor (SEE ILL18A). Only move the hands forward after you have tried to shoot the legs back from Lolasana. One day, you will surprise yourself! Jumping forward from Downward-Facing Dog works on the same principle and again I recommend that wherever you land, you keep hopping until you're through, rather than just sitting down. This will strengthen the upper body and *bandhas* and lead to eventual success. Finally, the best advice I was ever given when learning the *vinyasa* Jump-through was to allow the head to lead. In other words, as you jump back from sitting, the head actually goes in a forward direction and the legs moving back follow from that. Similarly, as you jump forward from Downward-Facing Dog, the head pulls

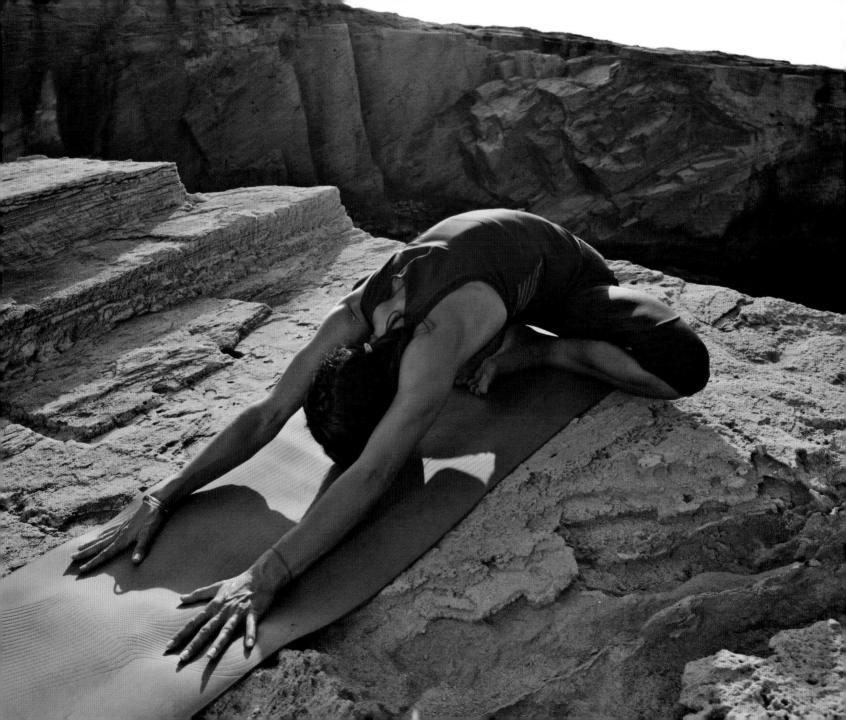

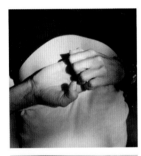

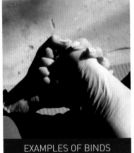

EXAMPLES OF BINDS

back and the legs move forward as a result. Humans tend to lead with their head, and the rest of the body follows suit. Understanding this phenomenon will help you master the half-*vinyasas* and other tricky movements.

To work the body in a more balanced manner and ensure a graceful dynamic, the linking laws in Quantum Yoga offer more alternatives. Here one posture informs the next. This entices you to pay attention and allows for true communication. It stills the mental turbulence by awakening spontaneous, creative and intuitive understanding. If attention is not paid, the balance in the sequence is lost, so this gives further impetus for conscious practice. As mentioned before, chose a certain common aspect of a group of poses as your leitmotif and allow that to be your linking mechanism. In this way you can sustain the flow, but reduce the amount of *vinyasa* Jump-throughs, thus focusing on quality rather than quantity.

JOINTS & BINDING

Many asana such as the *Marichiasana* group consist of binding the arms. The concept of *spanda*, or pulse, in the context of asana indicates that just as you extend out, so you must pull in. A lot of us hold tension in the joints and it is thus beneficial to work into them. However, we are mainly interested in stretching muscles, not ligaments, as the latter are designed to hold the joints in their place. Overextension of the ligaments will cause a decrease of stability in the joint,

which in turn can result in serious physical problems which often manifest in the simplest movements such as walking, running, lifting, carrying, climbing, and swimming. You should not have to sacrifice these basic activities to your asana practice. Partly due to the fact that I have pretty short arms (and legs, oh horror!) compared to the length of my torso, in order to bind, I have had to deliberately extend the arm out of the shoulder socket, then rotate it and finally wrap it around the leg in question, where it is then locked in place with the bind. Often this has been accompanied by an alarmingly loud clonking noise. Over time, it has caused instability in my shoulder. I have since become much more mindful of this and realize that even in an asana as familiar as the Downward-Facing Dog, I tend to extend out of the shoulder joint. Instead I now release back into it, while keeping the shoulders broad, which in turn actually serves to lengthen the neck.

A similar thing happened with the knee joint, but thankfully I have since managed to restore it through careful strengthening exercises and more mindfulness to the alignment. It is important to understand that the knee is only designed for a limited range of movement. The ankle and hip, on the other hand, can safely provide a circular motion. If the flexibility in these does not match the degree in which you are moving into your asana, the knee awkwardly positioned between the two will take the strain. Please be very mindful of this and proceed patiently. The knee has a lot to do with ego and eagerness to move forward. Remember the old saying, "Go slow, move far"!

BLOOD STOPPING, WIND LETTING AND PRESSURE POINTS

Students who are caught up in the idea that yoga is only for stretching often look at me in confusion and ask, "But what is this good for?" In yoga we work into far more than just the muscles. The entire body is made of spongy tissue suffused with blood and lymph. Any stagnation in the movement of blood through the body will trap toxins and impede the flow of oxygen and nutrients. When a part of the body is gently squashed and then released again, the blood is drained and then rushes back in with renewed vigor. At the beginning this may be very uncomfortable as there is great reluctance in the tissues to release toxins and waste products, but the more you practice, the less discomfort you will feel.

Many postures stimulate specific pressure points (marma), which allow the yogi to release blockages and thus transcend psycho-energetic restrictions held in these areas. Again this may be accompanied by discomfort, but like so many bitter medicines, discomfort may indicate that you are holding unnecessary issues in those areas. In *Janu Shirsasana B*, for example, the heel is placed against the perineum to stimulate *muladhara*, responsible for survival and basic instinct, and in *Janu Shirsasana C*, the heel does the same for *swadhistana*, the seat of sexuality and creativity. Be gentle on yourself, but

don't shirk away from sensation just because it is unusual and may even bring up unpleasant emotions and thoughts. If you don't work through it, you won't get rid of this discomfort.

I was recently asked to give a radio interview. One of the very first questions the presenter had prepared was, "What do you do if someone farts in your class?" It never ceases to amuse me just how this cliché gets perpetuated. "Well," I replied, "depending on the intensity, I may surreptitiously open the window, but mainly I just get on with it."

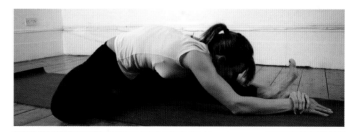

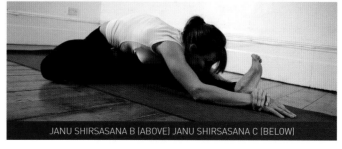

JANU SHIRSASANA B (ABOVE) JANU SHIRSASANA C (BELOW)

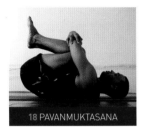

18 PAVANMUKTASANA

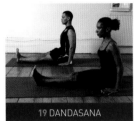

19 DANDASANA

As with the discomfort through constriction or pressure, so with letting wind, belching and profuse sweating: these naturally decrease with regular practice. It goes without saying that a practice that is specifically designed to rid you of waste will do so, until such time that a strong digestion has been established through the massaging of the organs and the strengthening of *jiva agni*, and the movement of the pranic winds or *vayus* has been regulated. "Better out than in," is what I say, although naturally in a class situation, it is advisable to be mindful of your fellow yogis. Don't be embarrassed though and, above all, persevere! The *Pavanmukti*, or wind-releasing group of asana, were specifically designed to facilitate the release of trapped wind (SEE ILL.18). In my experience, yoga regulates desires and will condition you to be drawn toward more sattvic, life-affirming and enlightening food and other consumables. Your practice and the well-being and clarity it affords become a priority and it is not even a matter of sacrifice, but a natural refinement of taste that will cause you to steer clear of activities that result in heaviness of body and sluggishness of mind.

CHOOSING YOUR FLOOR SEQUENCE

Dandasana:

Dandasana, the Staff or Rod pose, is the *Tadasana* of the seated poses. You should begin with it and come back to it after you have completed a set of poses. Here you sit upright, your body assembling itself along your spine, shoulders relaxed and hands placed by the side of your hips. Once you're seated on the floor, the challenge is to sustain good work in the legs, extending into the ball of the foot and pushing the heels and backs of the knees into the floor. Remember that muscles cannot stretch; they can only contract. Muscles work in pairs: as one side contracts, the other side gets stretched as a result. Therefore as the top of your leg tightens, the back of the legs release. The Standing Section comes before Floor Work to ensure this level of engagement and awareness in the legs, as this in turn protects your back. If in *Dandasana* it is hard for you to sit upright and hence there is a convex curve in the lumbar area, raise your seat by placing a block or cushion beneath it, which should help to flatten out the back (SEE ILL.19). In the neutral *Dandasana* position, the big toes are touching. Once you are doing variations with one leg, do not lose this correct angle of the foot remaining on the floor and keep the engagement in the straight leg! Just as the essence of *Tadasana* should be found in all your standing poses, so should you never lose *Dandasana* once you have come to the floor.

Forward-Bends:

Choose your floor sequence in accordance with your physiological needs and the energetic effect you want to achieve, and to prepare for your peak pose and stay within the theme you have elected. Should you have short hamstrings and tightness in the calves, frequent practice of forward bends is of course essential. Bear in mind that, as with the other types of postures, you will probably have done quite a bit of forward bending already as part of preceding groups. Nevertheless, having shifted your center of gravity to a seated position, you no longer need to contend with balance in the same way and can thus focus on refining and intensifying their effect.

Make sure to hinge from the hips and avoid rounding your back. Very often you are actually working deeper into the pose, by not coming so far down and instead focusing on the even extension of the spine. Remember that these are *forward* bends, not *down* bends. Hence, rather than aiming to get your face onto the knees, instead focus on extending the crown of your head forward. "Reach for China!" one of my first teachers used to instruct and this antiquated expression still rings in my ears as I wonder whether I'm facing east. *Paschimottanasana*, the simple seated forward-bend, means "intense west stretch," since the back of the body is referred to as its west. If you feel any lower back pain, it makes sense in forward-bends, whether standing or seated, to adopt a slightly wider stance of the legs.

Reaching and grabbing is the next aspect to be aware of. Often excessive pulling with the hands results in tightness in the shoulders, which causes the thoracic region to hunch up and

the neck to shorten. Postures should work the body evenly and stretching one area to the detriment of another is not in keeping with the wholeness we are cultivating through our yoga practice. I suggest you test yourself from time to time and do the *Mukta Hasta*, hands-free variation of the forward-bends. You will refine your asana by getting away from pulling. Instead tune into the effect of gravity, the softening that prana directed into the spine and back body with the help of the *bandhas* affords you, as well as once again the supporting effect that proper leg work has.

The correct *drishti*, or viewpoint, in forward-bends is a matter of debate among the yoga community. Yogis who suffer from tight shoulders and the *pitta* goal-oriented personality that often causes them should simply gaze down while keeping the chin in through *jalandhara bandha*, so that the neck is in an even line with the rest of the spine. This will further intensify the calming effect. *Kapha* personalities however could look forward, their gaze giving additional expression to the direction in which they are moving. *Vata*-types can do either, as long as they keep their eyes focused and don't fidget.

I have had many students for whom forward-bending is an intensely frustrating experience, as they feel they are "just not getting anywhere." Even after years they still can't touch their toes. Of course yoga isn't about touching your toes, but even the most enlightened mind may find this inability a bit disheartening. The way I work with these people is that I sometimes let the toes come to them. Connecting body parts and thus creating energy circuits can in itself be powerful. Therefore, why not just bend your knees sometimes! Even if you can touch your toes with straight legs, this softer approach has its place, and can give you more of an impetus to hinge from the hips and pull down the shoulders.

Forward-bends are stilling and inward-gazing asana. It is said that people who have problems with forward-bends have not dealt properly with their past. Whether you want to believe this or not, excessive tension held in the back body certainly indicates a lack of care for that which is behind you. Just because you can't see it, doesn't mean it's not there. Think about it!

Twists:

Many yogis dislike twists, but their cleansing and balancing effect is very significant. The main reason that twists are unpopular is that in the constriction of the twist, people find that their breathing is inhibited and a strangled feeling results. The truth is that this should give one even more reason to do twists. Although you have to make a special effort to draw the prana in, it is now being directed into unusual and often obscure parts of the body, those deep recesses that do not under normal circumstances get

supplied by prana. Remember that the nature of prana is cleansing and in this manner deep-seated toxins and negative emotions can get rooted out. So, twist away and here is how!

The stability of your foundation acquires added importance in a twist. Just as in the *Parivritta*, or rotated versions of the standing poses, you are holding your hips square, flattening the sacrum and stopping the pelvis from veering out to the side, so here you must be very clear from where you are generating the twist. As you twist to the right for example, if you allow the right hip to slide back and the left hip to move forward, you are not getting the twist into the spine, but generating it from the movement of the pelvis. Say you want to screw a cork out of a bottle. You would have to hold on tight, so that the bottle doesn't slide around in your hand. It is the same for your bum on the floor in the twist. The more grounded you can keep it, preserving the even alignment of the sitting bones, the deeper you will get into the spine.

Skillful twisting of the spine allows for rotational movement of the vertebrae, which ensures increased mobility and supports the release of blockages and tension. When you wring out a wet towel, not only do you twist it, you pull it too. So when twisting the spine, you need to be mindful not to scrunch up. Every time you inhale lengthen the spine, every time you exhale twist a little deeper. Once again work your body as a whole; twisting while shortening and hunching will not support the flow of prana.

It is advisable to twist in the direction of the natural movement of matter in the body first, which is to the right. Again it is the Quantum ethos to occasionally and consciously do it the other way around, and watch what effect that has. I often do this, particularly when I put the twist in as part of a flowing set and so far that has had no detrimental effects to body, brain or spirit!

Hip-Openers:

Just as it is important to cultivate the ability to work the legs as one unit, support the stability in the pelvis and keep the body aligned along its central axis, so it is also of utmost significance to increase one's range of movement safely and evenly and be able to spread out in all directions. For most people this expansive movement comes much more naturally in the arms, while the legs are relegated to the mere role of support and locomotion. Modern society's over-reliance on furniture means that most people lose the capacity to sit comfortably on the floor. If you look at the way a baby can easily sit cross-legged with an upright spine, you realize that the human body is actually designed to do so. Similarly, in societies that have maintained a more natural life, hips are open, backs strong, and the posture more upright. The familiar image of women effortlessly carrying large pots

of water on their head, demonstrates this ease in bodily alignment that many other cultures have lost.

Mastery of the Lotus Pose (SEE ILL.20) is one of the obvious aims of many yogis. The reason this is so desirable an objective is that *Padmasana* is possibly the best way to sit in meditation. The base is broad, the spine is held upright, ensuring that chakras and *nadis* are in perfect alignment. It promotes a relaxed alertness, and should the person fall asleep, they are likely to wake up from the sensation of toppling over, but without standing much danger of actually doing so. The Lotus furthermore symbolizes the clear mind and pure heart that the *sadhaka* (spiritual practitioner) maintains irrespective of circumstance, much like the pink-white lotus that grows even on the filthiest mud. Asana means "seat" and *Padmasana* is thus the ultimate seat, though there are many others that are suitable for meditation practice as described in the Meditation section below. It is of utmost importance when learning to do the Lotus to proceed with great patience and care, mainly with regards to protecting the knees. All cross-legged positions are hip-openers, as is *Baddha Konasana*, where the soles of the feet are placed together and the knees drop out to the side, and *Upavishta Konasana*, where the legs are spread at a right angle. By just holding the legs in this position, through gravity the hips will release over time. Naturally, this effect is increased if one bends forward, and here again, like with all

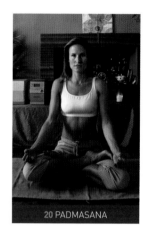

20 PADMASANA

forward-bends, one should be mindful not to hunch the spine or unnecessarily tighten the shoulders and neck. Pushing the legs or weighing them down in a hip-opening asana should only be done with the greatest care. If the knees are in any way vulnerable, it is advisable to place a support beneath them. Muscles actually release more easily when they are supported, rather than being suspended in mid-air.

Hips can also be opened with movements such as the "rocking the cradle." (SEE ILL.21) Here you are seated on the floor and cradle your bent leg, indeed rocking it like a baby. Bouncing movements such as the so-called Butterfly (moving the knees up and down in a seated *Baddha Konasana*) have

been proven to be counter-productive, as the muscles tense with each jerk. Supine hip openers such as the "threading the needle" are also nice alternatives. (SEE ILL.22) Lie on your back, bend your knees up and place the side of one foot against the opposite knee. Then thread your arm through the gap, the hands catching on the upright bent-leg knee and very gently pulling it towards the chest. Try to keep your head on the floor and the chin drawn in.

Once sufficient mobility in the hip joint has been established and the forward bend is strong, the yogi can proceed on to the leg-behind-head poses with all their manifold variations. Suryayantrasana (the Sun Dial, SEE ILL.23) is a good way to

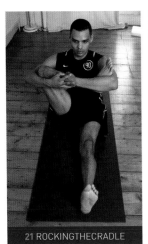
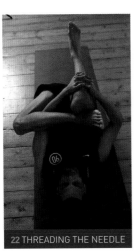
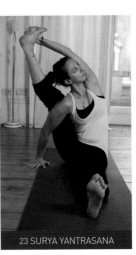
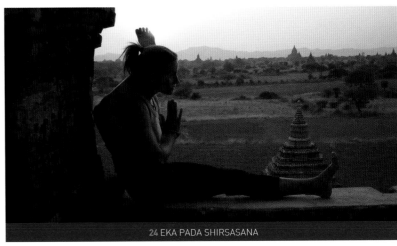

21 ROCKINGTHECRADLE

22 THREADING THE NEEDLE

23 SURYA YANTRASANA

24 EKA PADA SHIRSASANA

prepare for *Eka Pada Shirsasana* (One Leg Behind Head Pose, SEE ILL.24). Providing one proceeds slowly and maintains the steady, even *ujaii* breathing, working into this pose is relatively safe. It is only once you do actually manage to get the leg behind your head that you need to be mindful of the neck. The relative tightness in the hip can cause the neck to get strained. This can be avoided through *Jalandhara bandha*, as well as by firmly placing the palms beneath the jaw and thus supporting the head against the push of the leg. Through regular practice of this group of asana, not only will the hip eventually release sufficiently so that leg can comfortably remain behind the head, if one hasn't forced it, the neck will also get stronger. This is very useful for headstands (*Shirsasana*), shoulderstands (*Sarvangasana*), and backward rolls (*Chakrasana*), as well as to avoid such common causes of discomfort as whiplash and stiff neck.

THE HERO'S POSE VARIATIONS: A BOON FOR KNEES

It is advisable, especially if there is weakness in the knees, to follow hip-opening and Lotus variations with *Virasana* or variations thereof. The reason it is very hard for the knee to heal itself is that is receives little, if any, blood supply. The way to direct blood is to restrict its flow, and upon release, it will rush into this area as in *Virasana*, the Hero's pose, in which the leg is tucked under. Although the pose is good for knees, should there be an already existing injury, in particular in the

cruciate ligaments, great care needs to be taken. To come into the simple Hero's seat, kneel with your knees together and your feet hip-width apart. Press the fingertips into the backs of the knees to make space behind the joint and then carefully lower your sitting bones to the ground, whilst flattening the calves with the hands. Placing a folded belt tightly behind the knees increases *Virasana's* curative effect. Should the bum not reach the ground, place as many blocks as you need wide between the feet, so that the ankles are snug against its edge. Even if you are not using a support, make sure the ankles are hugging into the hips and the toes are pointing straight back. Do not yank the calves out to the side, as this over time can be detrimental to the knees. Instead flatten the calf by sliding the thumb or palm along it. *Virasana* can be used as a seat for meditation, you can go forward in it, or increase the stretch of the quadriceps by lying back. In *Supta Virasana*, the Supine Hero's Pose, make sure to squeeze the knees together and down towards the floor. If you feel you are pinching the lower

SUPTA VIRASANA

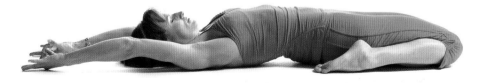

back either use bolsters under the spine as support, go into *Paryankasana* (Couch Pose) instead, or even just carefully arch back on your hands or elbows. Always work to your own capacity!

SHOULDER OPENERS

The neck is hugely affected by the mobility in the shoulders and due to office jobs and high stress levels, an increasing amount of people experience pain in this area. Postures such as *Gomukhasana* (Cow's Head Pose) where the hands are caught behind the back and others where the hands are placed in *namaste* prayer behind the back work directly into the shoulders. It is important to note here, though, that consciously keeping the shoulders away from the ears as the position and function of the arms changes, should promote relaxation in the shoulders in most every pose.

SPLITS

The splits really carry on from the standing poses and thus can be divided into two clear groups. The *Hanumanasana* (Monkey God Pose) or front splits, should consist of square hips, whereas *Samakonasana* (Great Angle Pose) or side splits, consist of flat hips. If this is respected and supported by good control in the legs, engagement of *mula bandha* to protect the groin (especially in side splits), *uddhiyana bandha* to protect the lumbar (especially in front splits), as well as steady *ujaii*

breathing, and providing one proceeds slowly and carefully, splits can be safely practiced even by beginners.

OTHER AND COMPOSITE POSES

There are as many asana as there are grains of sand. Every time you think you have mastered a pose, you will discover that there is another more difficult variation. This insight can be frustrating at times and yet it reveals one of the most precious aspects of spiritual practice. Being a yogi does not mean cementing a proud identity that boosts the ego. This can easily happen, as the body's appearance improves and the individual emits a strong and attractive presence. If one gets seduced by this power and exploits it for personal gain, it will trap and ultimately disappoint you, as your identification with and attachment to conditioned existence increases. The scriptures warn of the danger of being thrown off the path that should lead to freedom, if one gets carried away and misuses the siddhis or supernatural powers that yoga practice brings. When people are suddenly drawn to you, because they want something you have, such power presents itself. If you remember that yoga is not something you do or have, but a persistent practice and humble cultivation of a state of being that leads to the ultimate dissolution of the ego, you will steer clear of the pitfalls. Krishna's message to the handsome warrior-prince Arjuna was clear: to be a yogi means acting without desire for the fruits of one's actions, but

instead carrying out one's duty (*dharma*) with an attitude of
total dedication to the Supreme Principle.

FLOOR WORK POSES

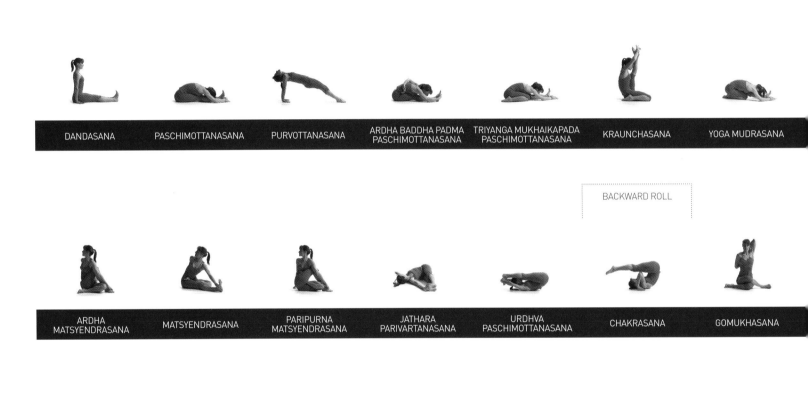

DANDASANA	PASCHIMOTTANASANA	PURVOTTANASANA	ARDHA BADDHA PADMA PASCHIMOTTANASANA	TRIYANGA MUKHAIKAPADA PASCHIMOTTANASANA	KRAUNCHASANA	YOGA MUDRASANA

BACKWARD ROLL

ARDHA MATSYENDRASANA	MATSYENDRASANA	PARIPURNA MATSYENDRASANA	JATHARA PARIVARTANASANA	URDHVA PASCHIMOTTANASANA	CHAKRASANA	GOMUKHASANA

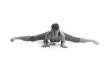

EKA PADA KAPOTASANA	HANUMANASANA	SAMAKONASANA	AKARNA DHANURASANA	SURYA YANTRASANA	EKA PADA SHIRSASANA	DWI PADA SHIRSASANA

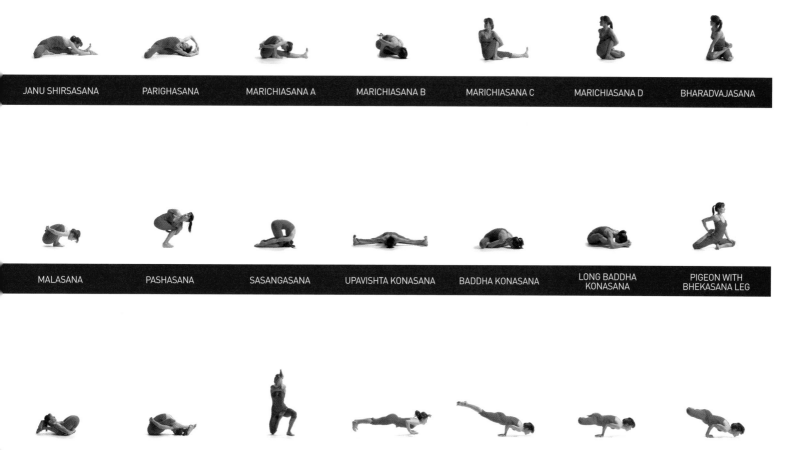

JANU SHIRSASANA   PARIGHASANA   MARICHIASANA A   MARICHIASANA B   MARICHIASANA C   MARICHIASANA D   BHARADVAJASANA

MALASANA   PASHASANA   SASANGASANA   UPAVISHTA KONASANA   BADDHA KONASANA   LONG BADDHA KONASANA   PIGEON WITH BHEKASANA LEG

YOGI NIDRASANA   KURMASANA   VATAYANASANA   NAKRASANA   MAYURASANA   PADMA MAYURASANA   PADMA HAMSASANA

06) ABDOMINALS

Separate abdominal exercises are only very rarely practiced as part of yoga sequences. The assumption in the *vinyasa*-based styles is that through the application of *mula* and *uddhiyana bandha*, the core is sufficiently strengthened. Also of course the aesthetic considerations of most yogis today do not feature in the traditional lore that valued correct energetic alignment over the "six-pack". Yet taking matters of current health requirements into consideration, most people's lifestyles are now largely sedentary and marked by a total reliance on furniture and overexposure to TV, computer and other screens. Therefore, for most people it makes sense to weave some specific abdominal exercises into a yoga sequence. The focus is on strengthening transverse abdominus, which means that rectus abdominus must be restrained. Abdominals need to be done with great care, particularly if the back is weak. This represents another catch-22: the back is protected by a strong core, but once there is pain or even injury, abdominal exercises must be approached very gently and mindfully. It is therefore best, despite most people's resistance to working directly into the "gut" area, to prevent such a situation early! Particularly with the energetic demands a serious yogi of any era makes on spiritual practice however, abdominal exercises should never lead to hardness, but tone and support posture conducive as much to strength as to stillness and joy.

Many modern health and fitness movements hone in on this current problem area, commonly referred to as "core." The results I see in students is that a certain control is often accompanied by an unnatural imbalance in the body and a sort of wooden rigidity. Unless the body is approached holistically, and placed in the service of a higher aim, the outcome will never serve the divine aspect of the being. Health for its own sake often backfires. This is because it does not keep the ego firmly yoked to a transformative intention. Without yoga, the ego often turns against itself and produces undesirable effects. Your breath as always is your monitor in the abdominals section, which people tend to either overdo or neglect entirely. The *ujaii* in its sound quality should indicate nonaggressive effort.

Any repetitions of exercises that resemble sit-ups must be done slowly and in synchronicity with the breath, while drawing the navel in and back and the pelvic floor up, with *uddhiyana* and *mula bandha*. This is the same with supine leg-raisers, where additional attention should be paid to keep the sacrum in firm contact with the floor throughout. In *Navasana* and variations thereon, it is tempting, just like in any forward-bend, to hunch the dorsal region, pull up the shoulders, and close off the chest. Instead, working with bent legs if you need to, draw the shoulders strongly down the back and really lift the sternum. This will afford you not only better balance, but

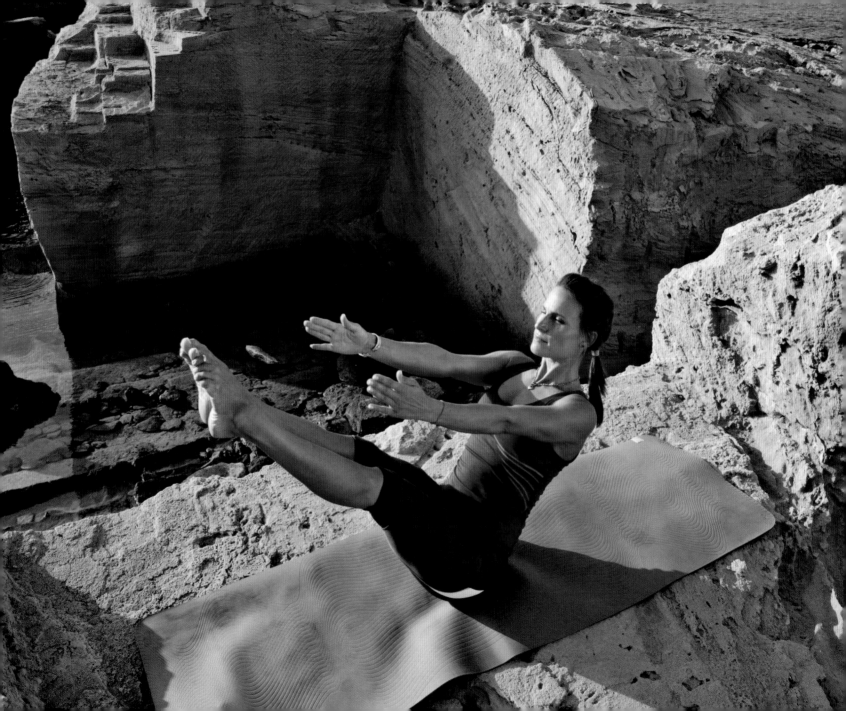

also space to breathe into. Just listen to the sound of the *ujaii* and you will recognize that its quality immediately improves!

If you practice Quantum Yoga in a skilled and conscious way, in terms of *bandha* and *ujaii* breath control, as well as structure and alignment principles, whether or not you add abdominal exercises as a separate group will be your choice. The abdominals have been placed before the backbends, so that after these muscles are contracted, they are lengthened again. The exception is that when an imbalance in *vata* has caused a flighty feeling and lack of integrity at the core, the openness and stimulation caused by backbends should ideally be "pulled together" again with abdominals, before one proceeds on to the inversions.

With the abdominals, we are after tone, not bulk. In view of the fact that Hatha Yoga is all about establishing the physical environment that facilitates a direct flow of prana along *sushumna nadi*, it is absolutely essential not to create the hardness of a six-pack, which actually hinders such an open and receptive posture. Shortening and hunching will decrease the yogi's ability to expand and receive prana on the inhalation and to sustain this expansion on the exhalation. It helps to think of the body four-dimensionally. Make space in the front, the back and the sides, while also embracing the realization that your energetic field expands beyond the confines of your physical self. Ultimately, of course, higher consciousness is infinite, the anandamaya kosha, your bliss body transcending all restrictions of time and space. (See Chapter 2, *Panchamaya Kosha*.)

ABDOMINAL POSES

NAVASANA   UBHAYA PADANGUSTHASANA   URDHVA MUKHA PASCHIMOTTANASANA   UPAVISHTA KONASANA   PRENKHASANA   BRAHMANDASANA   CLIVE'S EAGLE

GARBHA PINDASANA   VIKASITAKAMALASANA   INDONESIAN ABS

07) BACKBENDS

Backbends are primarily about opening the chest region and thus stimulating the *anahata* (heart) chakra. This is an area many of us protect and where much sadness can be stored. Even if you are one of those blessed persons, who consider themselves truly happy and fulfilled, everybody has experienced that root sadness of disconnection, when at a very early stage in life you learn to differentiate between good and bad, and the ego is formed. Initially, we are all born into a state of unconditional love and total acceptance. So when you open up to that possibility of no resistance again, strong sensations and, with it, raw feelings arise. Emotional outbursts and even tears are no rarity after backbends. These should not be held back. Yoga offers a safe environment in which to let go and rid yourself of unnecessary frustration that pertains to the past. Once you have stepped onto the path of yoga, you are returning to the essence from whence you sprang, but this time in a conscious way, which is the very reason this journey must be made. Why we get trapped in the first place by the great *maya-leela*, is the seeming paradox on which all of existence is based.

THE FUTURE

There is no doubt that backbends will take those yogis who are emotionally protective out of their comfort zone. It is said that limitations in backbends are an indication of a fear of the future. Certainly many of us have felt that reluctance to "expose" oneself in this manner, for a backbend often feels like you are letting your defenses down. The front of the body pertains primarily to the conscious self, the ego that moves forward. It is for this reason also that it is advisable to practice strong backbends only when a good foundation of asana experience has been established and then also to place this section into the second half of the sequence.

STRONG CORE—OPEN HEART

In order to undertake any physical, emotional, and spiritual realignment safely and to a positive effect, one must establish a strong core. In other words, the more solid your integrity, the easier it will be to truly open your heart without getting hurt or losing yourself in the process. The abdominals, pelvis, shoulders, thoracic region, and lungs all play part in this process. The spine is a natural s-shape. Almost everybody can backbend in the lumbar area, because it is already bending back anyway. Stand up and feel your lower back right now. Then move your hand up to the area between your shoulder blades; it is this convex area, where so many of us tend to hold tension, that needs to become concave in a backbend. Particularly flexible people will therefore have to learn to restrain the lumbar area in order to release the dorsal spine. If backbends are done without such awareness, perceived strengths will soon become weaknesses.

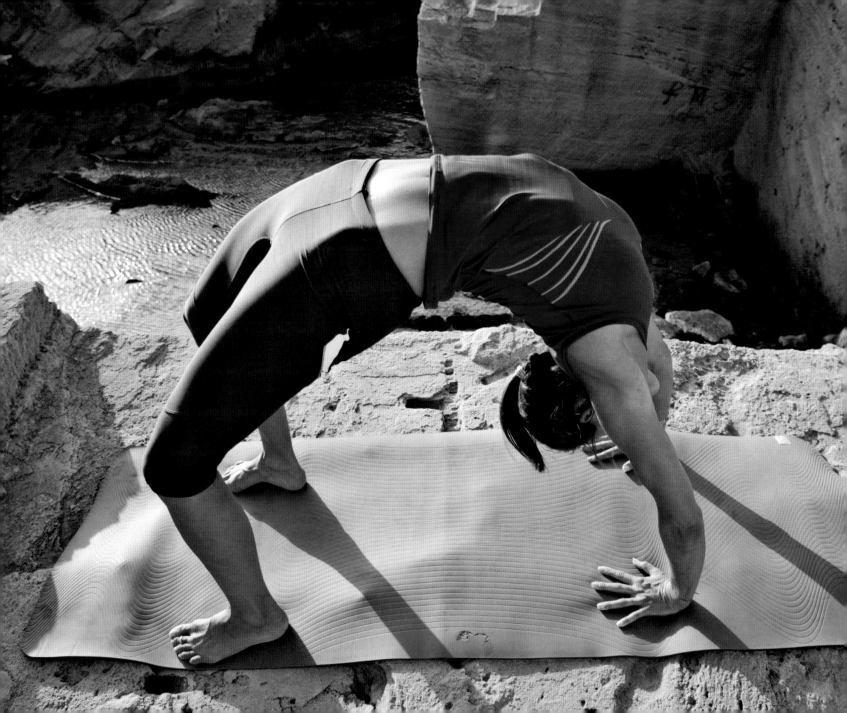

UPWARD BOW, DOWNWARD BOW AND UPRIGHT BOW

There are two basic types of backbends, those done on the belly, and those on the back. Then of course there are such variations as the Camel (*Ushtrasana*) and Full Pigeon (*Kapotasana*) that are done on the knees. No matter what type of backbend, one should always endeavor to turn what tends to be a push into more of a lift. There is a sacred geometry to backbends. Imagine a perfect arch, held up by two ball bearings at equal level. (SEE ILL.25) In order to establish this sacred geometry, the force applied by the arms and legs must be balanced.

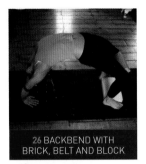

26 BACKBEND WITH BRICK, BELT AND BLOCK

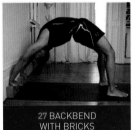

27 BACKBEND WITH BRICKS

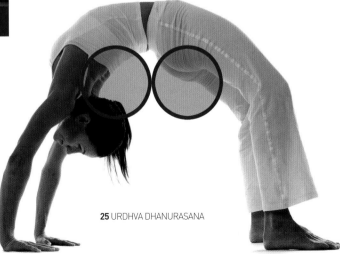

25 URDHVA DHANURASANA

As with any physical structure, the foundation of the pose will determine the quality of the entire asana. In the Upward Bow variations, such as what is commonly referred to as the Wheel, make sure that the feet are parallel, hip-width apart and not splaying. Really press the big-toe metatarsals into the ground and keep the knees directionally oriented towards each other. This will ensure that the lumbar area remains broad. Similarly, if the hands are used such in *Urdhva Dhanurasana*, press into the index finger knuckles and keep the elbows above the wrists throughout. This ensures breadth in the thoracic and shoulder region and avoids strain in the wrists. In certain cases where it is difficult to maintain this alignment, it is useful to use a looped belt just above the elbows. Similarly, a block can be placed between the feet to ensure their correct positioning and a brick between the knees will necessitate their squeezing together. (SEE ILL.26) Many individuals find it impossible to push off the ground and straighten the arms. In this case it is useful to use a pair of equally sized bricks placed lengthwise flush against the wall (SEE ILL.27). The palms are on the edge of the brick, with all fingers including thumbs pointing down. Not only does the increased height facilitate the lift-off, more importantly the fact that you have something to push against makes the ascent easier. If you have someone to assist you, they could also stand by your head with feet hip-width apart and slightly bent knees to protect their back, as you grab their ankles to facilitate the push-off (SEE ILL.28).

In *Setu Bandha Sarvangasana* (Shoulderstanding Bridge Pose), make sure, just as in a shoulderstand, that the shoulder blades are pulled in and you really are on your shoulders (SEE ILL.29). Interlock the fingers behind your back or grab your ankles, but only do the latter version if you manage to keep the soles of feet flat against the ground.

In the kneeling variations such as *Ushtrasana* (Camel), the knees should be placed hip-width apart and the feet need to be in line with the knees. Just like with splaying feet in *Urdhvh Dhanurasana*, so here if the knees slide apart and the feet together, you will jam your lower back. The legs remain engaged throughout, the pelvis moves forward, so that there is little or no weight in the hands. The positioning of the hands in *Ushtrasana* merely encourages the opening of the chest and heart region, further supported by the shoulder blades drawing flush against the back. In full *Kapotasana* (Pigeon), squeezing the elbows together and keeping the hands shoulder-width apart will also support the opening in the thoracic region (SEE ILL.30).

Backbends done lying facedown, such as *Dhanurasana* (Bow), *Bhujangasana* (Cobra), *Shalabhasana* (Locust), or *Bhekasana* (Frog) distinguish themselves by the fact that the body lifts off the floor, without the arms or legs pushing away from the ground. Even in the simple *Bhujangasana*, the feeling in the arms should be more of dragging the floor towards the body. Many people avoid this group of backbends like the plague, because they are hard, but often don't make you feel like you are going very far. Yet they are extremely useful in toning the back muscles! Yogis of a slimmer disposition may find it more pleasant to lay a folded towel or blanket as padding underneath the pelvis to protect the hipbones and what's in between. In *Dhanurasana* the upper and lower half of the body should lift up evenly and again the knees need to be squeezed towards each other to protect the lumbar region. In the simple version, I have my big toes touching to ensure that both sides are lifting evenly. In the version of *Dhanurasana* where you grab the inner ankles, flex the feet, and extend into the heels, check that you have turned the shoulders out, not in! In *Bhekasana*, commence by inhaling and lifting the upper body off the ground and on the out-breath twist the wrists and press down evenly through the balls of the hands. When done correctly, the legs are essentially in *Virasana* (Hero's Pose), and it is important not to press down on the feet unevenly, as this can cause injury in knees and ankles.

BHEKASANA

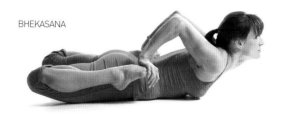

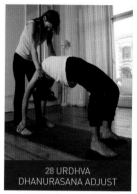

28 URDHVA DHANURASANA ADJUST

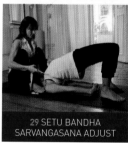

29 SETU BANDHA SARVANGASANA ADJUST

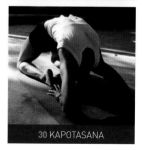

30 KAPOTASANA

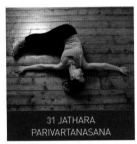

31 JATHARA
PARIVARTANASANA

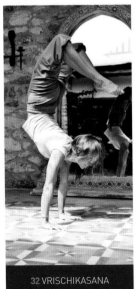

32 VRISCHIKASANA

BREATH AND TRANSITIONS

It is extremely important to be mindful of how you go in and out of a backbend, as it is on transition that most injuries occur. The smoother you move, the safer you will be. Monitor the quality of breath carefully, as it will clearly indicate whether or not you are being too forceful. Generally, beginners come into backbends on the out-breath, as this action requires strength and effort, which the exhalation supports. However, more experienced yogis may find that the inhalation takes you in more naturally, since a backbend is an expansive movement. The in-breath fills the lungs as the shoulder-blades pull down and the pelvis moves forward —all actions, in other words, that need to happen in the backbend anyway!

COUNTERPOSES: FORWARD-BENDS AND SUPINE TWISTS

A strong backbend session should be counterbalanced by a simple forward-bend such as *Paschimottasana*, but best left until the end of a series of backbends, so as not to confuse the spine. Also, supine twists such as *Jathara Parivartanasana* constitute appropriate counterposes (SEE ILL.31).

BACKBENDS IN OTHER SECTIONS

Some backbends such as *Matsyasana* (Fish Pose) are commonly taken into the finishing series. This is because they constitute a useful counter-pose to the shoulder-stand. Also,

as a result of opening *anahata* chakra in previous backbends, and the stimulation of *visuddhi* chakra in shoulder-stand, as well as the smooth line of energy and the clear *drishti* in the eyebrow center, the accrued pranic lifeforce and psychic energy is gathered in *ajna* chakra, the seat of wisdom at the third eye.

SCORPION AND OTHER BACKBEND INVERSIONS

Most of the time when we are backbending, we are working against gravity. Pushing up and away from it is always going to be harder than releasing back down to it. Once sufficient strength in the arms, balance, and core-control through *mula* and *uddhiyana bandha* have been established, releasing deeper into backbends in the inversions becomes possible. The skill here lies in releasing the feet down, in the same measure as you are lifting the head up (SEE ILL.32). Your *drishti* here, if you expand its definition of viewpoint to encompass intention and thus direction of movement, is the tips of your toes. Proceed slowly and mindfully, never excessively jamming the lumbar region and carefully monitoring the breath. Also, as with any inversion, make sure that there is nobody or nothing you could fall on. If you do lose balance, providing you have continued the deep, steady *ujaii* breathing which affords courage and prevents panic, you will land right on your feet. In my experience, once you have fallen, control becomes more difficult. Therefore practice *Vrischikasana* consistently, but never to excess in one session.

BACKBEND POSES

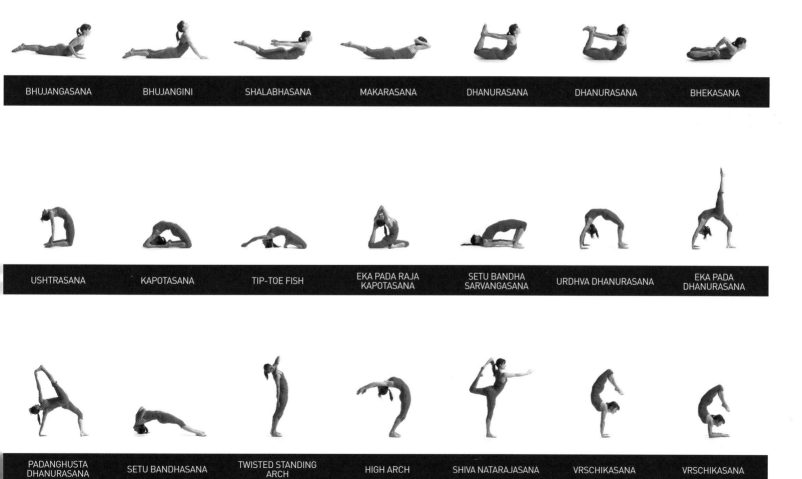

| BHUJANGASANA | BHUJANGINI | SHALABHASANA | MAKARASANA | DHANURASANA | DHANURASANA | BHEKASANA |

| USHTRASANA | KAPOTASANA | TIP-TOE FISH | EKA PADA RAJA KAPOTASANA | SETU BANDHA SARVANGASANA | URDHVA DHANURASANA | EKA PADA DHANURASANA |

| PADANGHUSTA DHANURASANA | SETU BANDHASANA | TWISTED STANDING ARCH | HIGH ARCH | SHIVA NATARAJASANA | VRSCHIKASANA | VRSCHIKASANA |

08) INVERSIONS

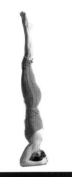

SHIRSASANA

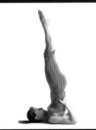

SARVAGASANA

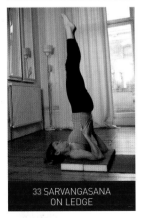

33 SARVANGASANA
ON LEDGE

Inversions are an integral part of all yoga practice. Turning your body upside-down literally has the effect of turning your view of the world around. The physical, psychological, and subtle energetic effects are far-reaching. It strengthens the immune system, aids the movement of blood and lymph, and supports the healthy functioning of all organs. By challenging your posture, structure, and alignment, you are therefore more aware of them. Inversions offer an altered view on reality and help one to pierce through to different realms of consciousness. For many practitioners, going upside-down means facing their greatest fear. To know that the head and thus the brain can become a structural support puts things further into perspective. Gravity exerts its force not merely on the material body, but also aids the upward energetic flow of prana. Tradition even has it that going upside-down temporarily halts the *amrit* (nectar of immortality that is said to drip from the *bindu*, the source-point at the pineal gland) from being consumed by the gastric fire.

The basic finishing inversions are *Shirsasana* (Headstand) and *Sarvangasana* (Shoulderstand). These are further subdivided by their *salamba* (supported) and *niralamba* (unsupported) variations. Moon-day girls should not go upside-down for any extended period of time, but practice *Supta Baddha Konasana* or *Upavishta Konasana* instead. (See *Menstrual Practice and the Moon Cycle* section, Chapter 5, for detailed explanation).

The effect of *Sarvangasana* (Shoulderstand) is stilling and balances *vissudhi* (throat) chakra. It also strengthens the thyroid gland and turns the *drishti* to the navel, which further calms the system. Take your time when coming into shoulderstand. Many people's shoulders are naturally turned forward. Therefore, in order to really get onto the tops of the shoulders, it helps to come into *Halasana* (Plow) first, interlock the fingers and carefully wiggle onto the tops of the shoulders, always of course safeguarding the neck. To stop the elbows from sliding back together, one can use a shoulder-width looped belt around the arms, placed just above the elbows. Persons who have a fragile neck may prefer to place the shoulders slightly raised up on a folded blanket or four blocks wrapped into the yoga mat to avoid them sliding apart. (SEE ILL.33) Keep a little extra space from the edge, as your shoulders will roll back as you come up. The head remains on the floor and therefore there is no direct pressure on the neck. Beware as you raise the legs up if you are not used to this, as you will feel much higher and you do not want to end up toppling over in surprise. Many styles recommend that students always use this elevation, but do note that of course since the chin-lock is somewhat reduced, the intensity of the stimulation of the thyroid gland on a physical level and that of *vissudhi* chakra on an energetic level is somewhat reduced. Nevertheless, if you have a fragile neck, it is well worth setting the posture up in this way.

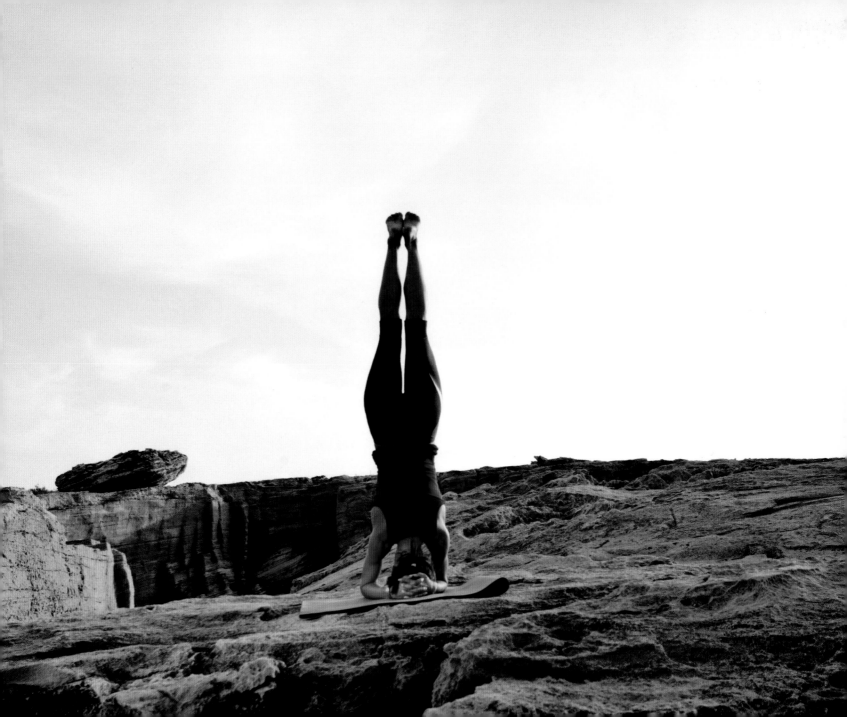

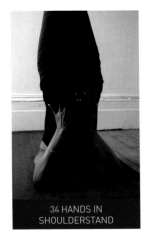

34 HANDS IN SHOULDERSTAND

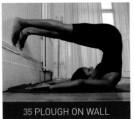

35 PLOUGH ON WALL

In *Salamba Sarvangasa*, where the palms are supporting the back's upright position, ideally all fingers should be in line and pointing up, so that the hands act like an upright ledge. (SEE ILL.34) In this way, the weight is evenly distributed along the surface of the palm, which constitutes an even structural support, rather than the fingers awkwardly grabbing the flesh, which strains wrists and tenses shoulders. Of course, with growing core strength, good legwork and strong *ujaii* breath, the body is able to hold itself upright without much support.

It is at this point that the *niralamba* variations are introduced. Begin by laying the arms alongside the head on the floor, so there is still some form of support. If you are nervous to change the positioning of the arms when already in shoulder-stand, begin with a Plow (*Halasana*) in which the arms are in this position, and lift the legs up from there (SEE ILL.35). Once you are confident in this, try the full *Niralamba Sarvangasana*, with the arms stretching up alongside the body, or in front with palms facing the thighs. As with the legs, so with the

arms, the more you radiate those fingertips confidently up to the sky, the easier it will become to hold yourself upright. Especially once it is easy for you, *niralamba* should not be regarded as a replacement for *Salamba Savangasana*, as the latter is actually more effective at opening the shoulders.

As mentioned before in the *Backbend* section, *Sarvangasana* is often followed by *Matsyasana* (Fish, SEE ILL.36) or *Paryankasana* (Couch) as a counterpose. In the Ashtanga finishing sequence, *Matsyasana* is followed by *Uttana Padasana* (Upwardly Extended Leg Pose), which is useful in strengthening the core before the headstand (in which many yogis tend to collapse the lumbar and bulge out the belly). The latter however should not be done if there is already pain in the lower back. (See *Abdominals* section, Chapter 3.) Being a backbend, *Matsyasana* is of course stimulating, so if the practitioner wants to ensure deep relaxation and maximize the stilling effect of their Quantum Yoga practice, it is more advisable to roll from the shoulderstand slowly, vertebra by vertebra, straight into

36 MATSYASANA

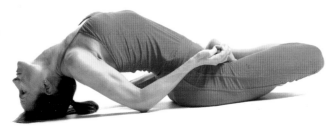

37 BALASANA

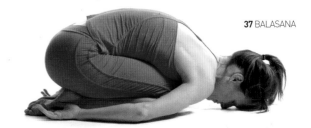

Savasana. Conversely, if we are consciously working through the subtle energetic alignment of the body, *Matsyasana* with its intense *drishti* in *ajna* chakra makes perfect sense.

Shirsasana is regarded in the scriptures as the "king of asana" and is focusing, energising, and when done correctly, stabilizes and aligns the entire body. It stimulates *sahasrara* (crown) chakra, which as it lies outside of the physical confines of the body, brings an elevated level of awareness to the yogi. *Shirsasana* thus establishes a direct connection to the subtle body. More than any other inversion, it supports the upward flow of prana along *sushumna nadi* and with it the ultimate awakening of kundalini shakti. *Shirsasana* constitutes the straightest vertical line, the dynamic inversions (handstand and forearm balance) always containing a degree of backbend. This also means that blood flows into the head and pressure builds up in the brain. Therefore make sure to always hold *Balasana* (Child's Pose, SEE ILL. 37) after a long-held headstand! Cases of strokes have been reported after headstand, so please approach this powerful asana with respect. In the Ashtanga Intermediate series seven headstands are done in succession, dropping straight into *Chatwari* (Press-Up Position) and putting a half-*vinyasa* in between, and in the Advanced Series this routine becomes even more pertinent. More experienced yogis whose bodies are accustomed to inversions, can do this without a problem,

especially if, as in this case, the headstand is not held for any more than five breaths. Like with any other aspect of yoga practice, mindfulness is key. If you pay attention to how the body feels, monitor the quality of your breath, and cultivate smooth transitions in and out of postures, responding accordingly, you will reap great benefits from this powerful pose. It is one of my personal favorites and I especially enjoy it on a beach at sunset, watching the radiant ball rise into the ocean, casting its fiery rays, as though someone had just thrown a bucket of gold across the water that is now transformed into my pink sky.

FEET: POINT OR FLEX?

Yogis are renowned for their obsession with feet and as they are at the top in inversions, their importance here moves even more into the foreground. In the spirit of Quantum Yoga, the only hard-and-fast rule with feet is that they should be conscious and alive. Pointing the toes (actually also referred to as "plantara flexion") is very effective in providing extra lift, causing the whole body to pull away from gravity. Flexing the feet (or "dorsiflexion") and extending into the heels tends to have the effect of flattening the body, so it is very helpful for the bendy types, who find it hard to find the balance due to an overly flexible lower back and lack of core. The golden middle way is to engage the feet so that they curiously resemble those of a Barbie doll. The extension comes from the center, runs along the inner thigh and is out through the ball of the foot. This footwork in turn cultivates a level of awareness that when standing upright translates into an avoidance of the all-too-common collapsing of weight onto the outer back heel. Take a look at the soles of your shoes; their wear should give you a good indication of your personal tendency.

ORDER

In the Ashtanga versus the Iyengar tradition, there is a big debate as to which one of the two finishing asana, Shoulderstand or Headstand, should come first. I remember being severely told off at the Iyengar Institute in Pune for getting it wrong. Really neither way is "wrong" as it all depends on what effect you are aiming to produce, as well as what kind of practice preceded your finishing inversions. If you have done a lot of strong backbends, it is an evening session and you want to ensure sound sleep, or you simply feel generally unsettled, definitely complete your Quantum Yoga practice with a long held shoulder-stand. Should you on the other hand be working more on a subtle energetic level towards a consolidation of psychic energy at the third eye and finally the expression of this cosmic union at the crown chakra, completing your practice with *Shirsasana* makes much more sense. There are yet other traditions, such as Shivananda, where *Shirsasana* and *Sarvangasana* are placed directly after the *Suryanmaskara*, and *Trikonasana* is

done last. All traditions are equally valid in their own right. Quantum Yoga encourages you to safely explore the effects of the various asana and learn to make conscious and informed decisions pertaining to your personal practice. This will in time allow you to speed up your progress immensely, so that the initial goal of total well-being and inner peace, and perhaps even the ultimate aim of union with the Absolute may not seem quite as out of reach as they once appeared. You are the master of your destiny, because you impersonate a unique manifestation of the divine!

INVERTED POSES

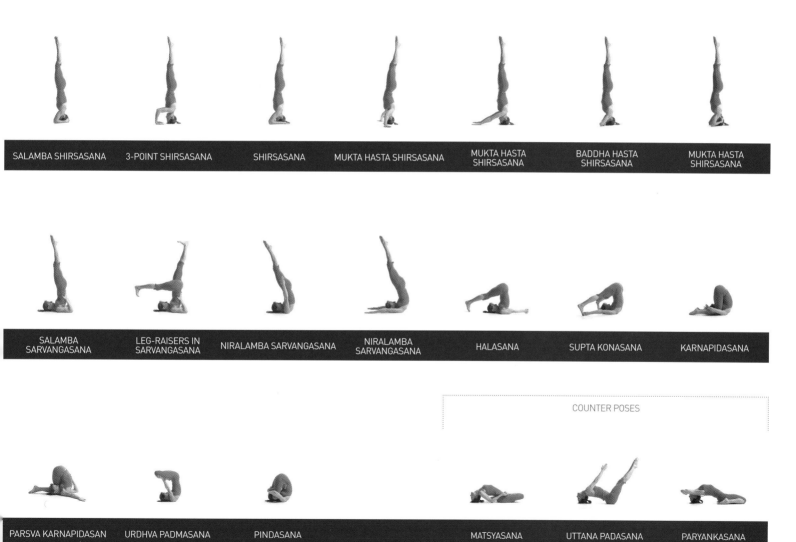

| SALAMBA SHIRSASANA | 3-POINT SHIRSASANA | SHIRSASANA | MUKTA HASTA SHIRSASANA | MUKTA HASTA SHIRSASANA | BADDHA HASTA SHIRSASANA | MUKTA HASTA SHIRSASANA |

| SALAMBA SARVANGASANA | LEG-RAISERS IN SARVANGASANA | NIRALAMBA SARVANGASANA | NIRALAMBA SARVANGASANA | HALASANA | SUPTA KONASANA | KARNAPIDASANA |

COUNTER POSES

| PARSVA KARNAPIDASAN | URDHVA PADMASANA | PINDASANA | MATSYASANA | UTTANA PADASANA | PARYANKASANA |

09) RELAXATION

Savasana, or Corpse Pose, represents a state of deep relaxation, yet total awareness. This disciplined relaxation should not be mistaken for sleep. It is conscious pure being, at one with the entirety of existence. The less you do here, the more effective the process of healing set up by the preceding practice will be! In fact the state of *Savasana* is akarmic. *Karma* literally means "action" and action is threefold: physical, mental, or somnial. The Corpse Pose is none of these. It is important to clearly mark the entry into *Savasana* either by a deep sighing exhalation through the mouth, a total tensing and then releasing of all the muscles in the body, or rapid breathing while lifting the body off the ground such as in *Utpluthih*. The *bandhas* must be consciously "unlocked" to soften the inner body. The breath returns from *ujaii* to relaxed soundless abdominal breathing. *Savasana* represents a dissolution into the totality of being and yet an integration of all of existence into oneself. One surrenders the material body, melting into the earth and dissolving into the air all around. It is a return to the elements. Imagining oneself as a corpse may strike many people as a rather unattractive notion, but if death means handing over the body so that the spirit returns to its source, in Savasana we really are dipping into Shiva's transformative field.

The obvious option in *Savasana* is to be in a state of silence, enveloped only by the sound of your breath and the song of nature. You expand into the vast macrocosm of universal interconnection. In particularly deep states of absorption, you may encounter a soft hum, a deep sweet sizzling sound that emanates from within. It is rare that the unstruck sound, or nadam, reveals itself at this stage, so most of the time your encounter here is within. Here you are integrating deep levels of self-perception into your consciousness. You sense the inner rumblings of the organs, the buzz of sanguine energy pulsing through your veins and *nadis*, and the rhythmic throng of your heartbeat. You are hearing life. Sometimes you can play with going in and out of this microcosmic state to a macrocosmic state at will.

Music of course can be very useful in aiding relaxation, as long as it is appropriately chosen. This is especially the case if you live in an urban environment and there is noise from traffic or the likes. Visualizations can be very useful here too. I often gently suggest to my students when in *Savasana* to visualize the prana in their body as a pinkish hue enveloping every single cell in its benevolent embrace. Then I describe the *sushumna nadi* as a line of golden energy flowing through the center of the body, like a radiant ray of light. In the head there is a cool bluish void. Not a nihilistic emptiness, but a space that holds infinite potential, which we have chosen to keep in a state of total rest for the time being.

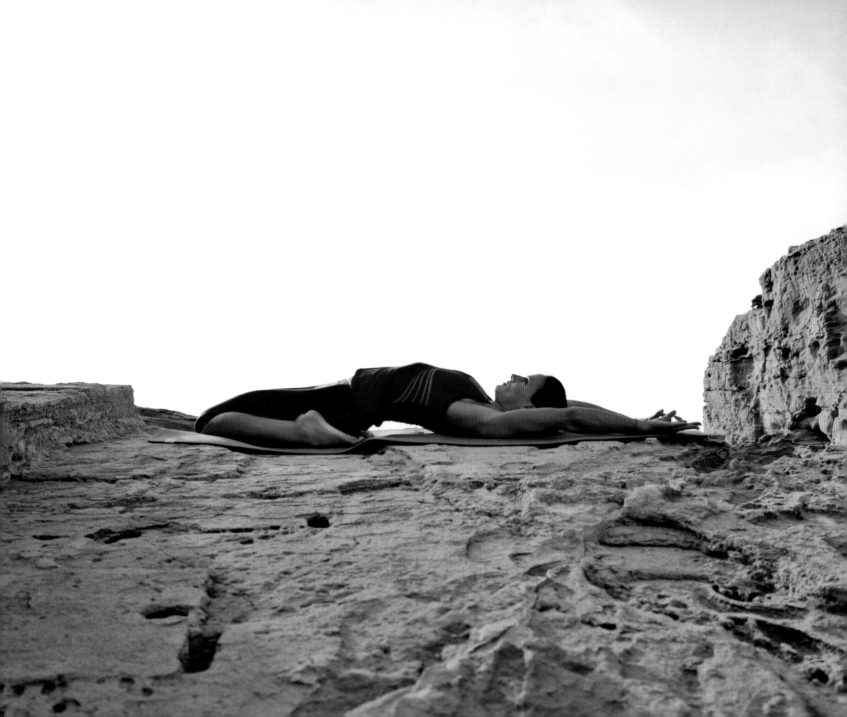

The other possibility, especially with a view to ensure the physical relaxation of all parts, is to scan the body slowly from the toes right up to the crown of the head, really feeling one's way deeply right into the microcosm of the cells. True relaxation needs to be patiently practiced and carefully observed, as most of us unconsciously hold tension even when we think we are letting go. I used to and still sometimes do have (try not to laugh here!) a tense right buttock, which I'd have to consciously unclench; otherwise it could go an entire *Savasana* unnoticed. It is crucial to become aware of these things, as they are usually indications of your body compensating for some weakness, but in the process aggravating the imbalance. Once such a phenomenon has been noted, it can then be carefully addressed in the next asana session. The Quantum Method will allow you to construct a sequence for this purpose.

Take yourself out of *Savasana* slowly, by first wiggling fingers and toes to come back to your physical self. Then bend your knees and roll onto your right-hand side. From there gently push yourself up to sitting. Make sure not to jerk into an upright position. Particularly after a strong asana session, in which the body will have been stretched and loosened and then relaxed, it is not advisable to suddenly jolt the muscles into a contraction. Move like a baby until you have found a comfortable upright position. Now you are ready to

either seize the day or night, or go into meditation. With the constraints most of us have on our time, we only rarely find the occasion to sit for meditation, but please do remember that ultimately asana practice was designed to support a steady and comfortable seat from which to access more elevated states of consciousness by bringing the mind to a state of total stillness.

Savasana is not the only relaxation pose. Particularly if you have done a *pitta*-regulating practice and kept the energetic expenditure at an even keel, it may not be necessary to go into corpse, as the system has not been hyped up. Sometimes, I go straight into meditation in *Padmasana* (Lotus), but follow this by *Supta Virasana* (Supine Hero's Pose) to counterbalance the stretch in the legs. Also, if I follow a finishing headstand with a long-held *Balasana* (Child's Pose), and from there I simply go into meditation in *Virasana* (Hero's Pose).

RELAXATION POSES

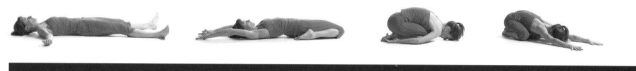

SAVASANA	SUPTA VIRASANA	BALASANA	BALASANA

MEDITATION POSES

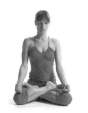
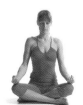
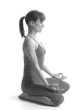
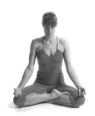
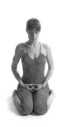
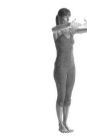

PADMASANA	SUKHASANA	BADRASANA	SIDDHASANA	VIRASANA	HUGGING A TREE

10) MEDITATION

Quantum Yoga, when done in the true spirit of expansion of consciousness and a quest for truth, represents a dynamic form of meditation, where the yogi becomes one with the practice. A state of absorption (dhyana) in movement is thus cultivated. Nevertheless yoga asana was primarily designed to ensure that the practitioner can sit steadily and at ease in meditation. It would therefore be a shame not to do so regularly. Listed below are a few simple guidelines and practices that will suffice in establishing a regular seated meditation.

OBJECT OF FOCUS

In meditation we cultivate one-pointed focus in order to reach a state of cosmic consciousness. There is always this dichotomy in yoga and all genuine mystical traditions, that of closing in on one point till all thought dissolves and the mind slips through that loophole into infinity.

Choose an object or point of focus and stay with it. This supports dharana (concentration), and leads to dhyana (absorption). Most meditation is done with the eyes closed, so that the object of focus is internal. This is not the only way though, and especially if you are tired or *kapha* is unbalanced, you may want to keep your eyes open and on a single point, or perhaps on a flower, an icon, a yantra, or the flame of a candle. (See Chapter 5 for details.)

Nevertheless, from what I have gathered, most people's minds are excessively busy and keeping the eyes closed offers less distractions. The third eye (*ajna* chakra) represents a powerful psychic center and using this as an internal focal point, will leave you with a truly cosmic feeling. This is also referred to as shambhavi mudra, as it "seals" a specific energy circuit. Hence the powerful effect, but please bear in mind again that the real challenge is to avoid getting carried away with the "trippy" feelings and psychedelic visions that prolonged focus in *ajna* chakra can easily lead to. Focus in the heart center (*anahata* chakra) on the other hand, will support a warm feeling of loving compassion.

POSTURE IN MEDITATION

The ideal posture for meditation practice is *Padmasana*, the Lotus Pose. Alternatively, if the hips are still tight, *Sukhasana* (Pleasant Pose) or *Siddhasana* (Perfect Pose or Adept's Seat) are fine as well. When the hips or knees begin to ache, you can vary these cross-legged positions by tucking the legs under in *Virasana* (Hero's Pose) or *Badrasana* (Noble Pose), where the knees are wider and you are sitting in the cradle of your feet. It is better to use a prop (like a cushion or block) to elevate your sitting bones off the floor or support your knees than to be so uncomfortable that you cannot concentrate. Conversely, if you are constantly busy trying to avoid any form of discomfort, sitting still will be very difficult, no matter how

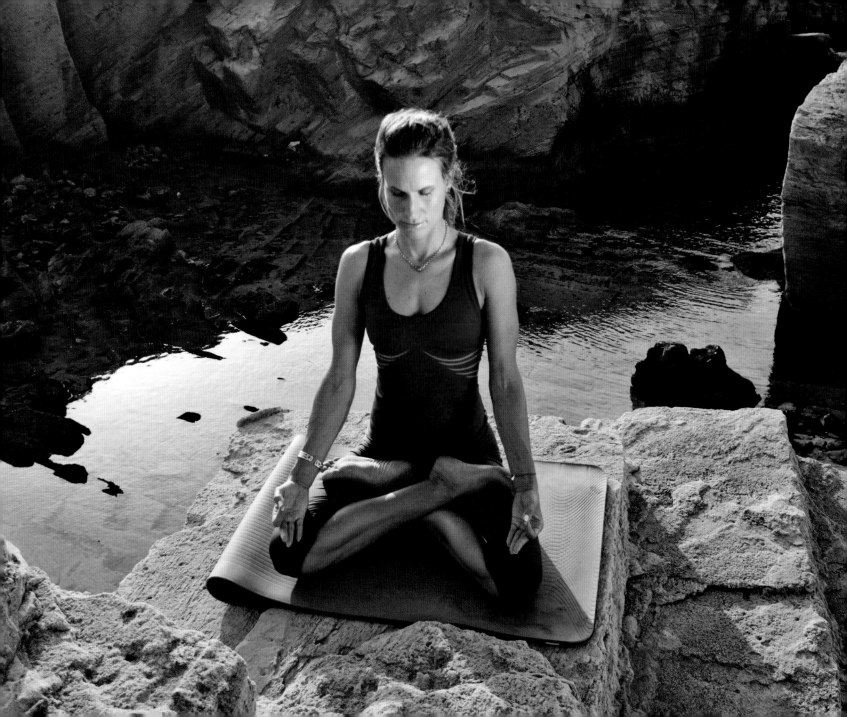

well-prepared and supported by props you are. In my early years of sadhana, at a particularly arduous retreat, one fellow yogi who noticed my fidgeting took me aside and gave me one of the best pieces of advice I have ever had. "Have you noticed that when you change your position in meditation, a few moments later you're uncomfortable again?" You bet I had! "So you might as well just stay where you are," he went on to suggest. If you sit still, you soon come to realize that sensations, just like everything else in this fluctuating world, change all the time. The most unbearable ache can give way to a positively pleasant numbness; a lovely tingle can suddenly become an annoying itch. Freedom is being able to watch all this and know that your true divine self is totally unaffected by it. In themselves, these are just empty sensations before we label them as good or bad and then go about reacting.

Naturally, if the body is too weak or due to injury or birth defects it is not possible to sit upright, meditation can be done sitting on a chair, or even lying down as well. There are also forms of meditation that create energetic fields to hold your focus, such as "hugging the tree" (see photo chart), or others that invite awareness in ordinary movements such as walking meditation.

CASE STUDY: "MINDFULNESS IN BREATHING"

This mental exercise is done in four distinct stages, each of which should be allocated approximately the same amount of time. Be realistic and don't set the goalpost too high! Even just sitting still for twelve minutes can seem like an eternity if you have never attempted meditation before. You count the breath up to ten and back down to one again, beginning with short intervals (inhale *one*, exhale *two*, inhale *three*, etc.) and then widening them (inhale-exhale *one*, inhale-exhale *two*, inhale-exhale *three*, etc.). The next stage is to observe the sensations at the tip of the nose resulting from the flow of breath. Finally, you follow the breath, as it enters and spreads through the microcosm of the body, and then as it exits and expands into infinity. Obviously the mind cannot wrap itself around infinity! That is how, in this Buddhist exercise, the mind is "tricked" into realizing a state of cosmic consciousness. However, this also means that it is much more likely to lose itself in thought again, in which case go back to the last step or even the one before, and patiently start again.

Even when yoked to a single point (*ekagrata*), the thoughts of "monkey mind" will grasp for any possible branch to be distracted, not to mention the senses always grappling for outer stimuli. You hear a sound, and the eyes can't resist sneaking a peak to investigate where it came from. And even if you resist those outer temptations, the mind throws up memories, projects into the future, remembers, plans, and fantasizes. Entire movies are spun out in your mind, when actually all you wanted was to *not think*! Getting annoyed and ordering the mind to stop just constitutes another thought. Meditation is challenging, and that is because your mind was designed to think—much like an organ doing its function regardless of your decisions.

Therefore, without anger or impatience, lovingly guide your attention, again and again, back to the chosen focal point. Your higher intellect (*buddhi*), though still a faculty of the mind (*manas*), does not get carried away with emotional charges and instead keeps things simple. With time, the gaps between the thoughts will widen and it is here that you will find your true freedom, lasting peace and unconditional bliss. The mind can be likened to a body of water: turbulent ripples cutting across its surface from all directions, smashing into each other, and incessantly perpetuating more movement (*chitta-vrtti*). When that ocean of thought finally comes to a state of stillness, it will become like a mirror and reflect back pure consciousness.

Samadhi, *nirvana*, *moksha*, *kaivalya*, *enlightenment*—whatever you may want to call it—is not a place or reward, nor is it a goal or achievement. It is a simple state of consciousness that is always there at the base of your ever-fluctuating thought processes. Although disciplined and consistent yoga practice will lead to this liberated state, one can also be propelled into it suddenly and unexpectedly. Faith—holding the conviction that with practice, you are taking yourself closer to liberation—is important. Yet ultimately one must free oneself from goal-oriented thinking altogether. The Taoists speak of the desire to not desire, because if you strive for the enlightened state as though it were something you want to master or conquer, you are being guided by the ego, and this will only take you further into a dualistic experience of reality.

My experience is that when you sit in meditation, the best you can do is to observe your thoughts, without judgement or analysis. Be relaxed and alert. The more loving and patient you can be with yourself, always stirring your attention back to the object of focus, unwavering but never rigid, the sooner you will find that you enjoy these periods of inner contemplation. That which you enjoy, you will keep doing. And if you keep finding time to sit in meditation, you will eventually pierce through to that indescribable sanctuary of ecstatic serenity, where every inkling of your being is saturated with wonder and you realize once and for always that all of existence is generated by love.

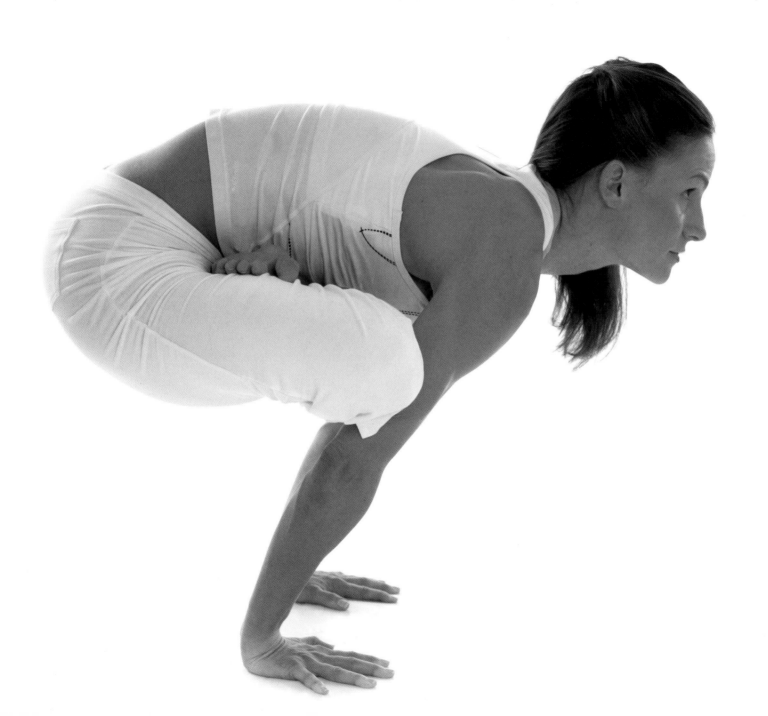

CHAPTER FOUR
THE THREE BASIC
QUANTUM SEQUENCES

BIRDS

A VATA-REGULATING YOGA SEQUENCE IN THE QUANTUM METHOD

Yoga is the process of revealing the true nature of reality, acknowledging the divine essence that runs through all existence, and reclaiming our natural state of freedom. Yoga transforms us by clearing away energetic and psychic obstacles that keep us from realizing our personal potential, while embracing the fundamental oneness of being. Practicing asana and *vinyasa* helps the body to assume its true shape, clearing its energy-channels and allowing prana to flow harmoniously. The Birds Sequence regulates *vata*, the Ayurvedic *dosha* of air, and thus teaches grounding and a conscious incorporation of the force of gravity to imbue the practice with the lightness and grace this lofty disposition longs for, while preserving safety and steadiness. This sequence is designed to liberate and empower, incorporating asanas named after birds: *Bakasana*, *Garudasana*, and *Kapotasana*. These postures cultivate qualities essential in asserting our freedom: balance and concentration, a strong steady connection to the earth, integrity at our core, and an open and joyful heart. The sequence peaks with *Eka Pada Raja Kapotasana*, the One-Legged King Pigeon Pose. Within this pigeon lies the heart of a dove—the symbol of the deep inner peace cultivated through the practice of yoga. From this sanctuary of inner peace universal harmony will become manifest.

The theme of Birds is freedom. In the spiritual context this ultimately means freedom from the cage that the mind creates for us. This bondage is the result of a misidentification with our inner turbulence, which in itself only reflects the outer reality, as perceived by the senses, which is in a perpetual state of flux. In this dualistic mode of consciousness, there can be no peace, no stillness, no true balance, as the only thing that is permanent is change. Our thoughts embroil us, firing off emotions, and we are caught in a state of frustration, trying to find fulfilment, meaning, true happiness and stability in a world that keeps disappointing us. Freedom therefore exists only when we realize that ultimate reality is what we experience when we learn to control the mind, slow down and ultimately stop the thoughts. In this state our true blissful nature emerges, and we learn to access this inner sanctuary at will.

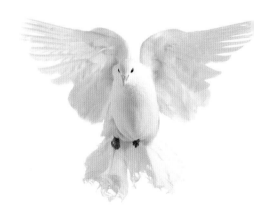

HEROES
A PITTA-REGULATING YOGA SEQUENCE IN THE QUANTUM METHOD

Yoga represents the methods and means that lead to a direct experience of the divine essence of reality. This sacred practice is approached with focus and discipline, referred to as *tapas*, or spiritual fervor, while at the same time cultivating joy and encouraging playfulness. The root "tap" denotes heat and the Heroes Sequence is designed to deal with our fiery nature, referred to as *pitta* in Ayurveda, and cool our passionate temper while channeling this potent energy in a sustainable manner so it results in true strength. The body is purified through the heat generated from asana-*vinyasa* in conjunction with *ujaii pranayama*. The mind in turn is stilled and one's general disposition becomes cool and clear. A hero is neither aggressive nor reluctant to act, but instead masters the skill of balancing force with yielding. This sequence incorporates many variations on the Hero's Pose (*Virasana*) and is designed to smoothly strengthen every part of one's being. Thus it creates a steady platform from which to embrace our true form, realize our creative potential and bravely express our wild and loving nature. The state of yoga or union is founded on the realization that we are all connected as One and that therefore everything we do matters. Quantum Yoga encourages you to recognize this eternal truth and live by it.

The Hereos Sequence represents a celebration of the female aspect of reality, often referred to as Shakti, the generative and creative power contained in nature. It takes true strength to avoid being seduced by the power that yoga undoubtedly gifts you. By instead continuously interacting with one's more vulnerable sides and seeking ways to cultivate balance and harmony, inner and, ultimately, universal peace can be coupled with power to reach perfection—the postures in Heroes reflect this truth. The Heroes sequence includes *bija* mantras, primordial sounds of nature or "seed sounds" to harmonize the energy in each chakra, visualization aids, as well as cooling breathing exercises that increase lung capacity.

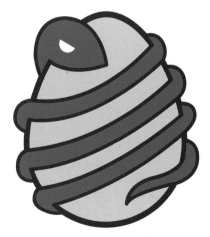

LOTUS MANDALA
A KAPHA-REGULATING YOGA SEQUENCE IN THE QUANTUM METHOD

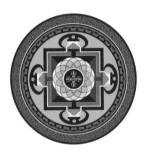

Yoga increases prana—the life force that brings vitality, health, and happiness to the individual. Often through a sedentary lifestyle, lack of inspiration, and consumption of unhealthy foods, a person feels heavy, toxic, and depressed. In Ayurveda this would be viewed as an imbalance in *kapha*, the biological humor of earth/water. This means that an asana practice that maximizes the vinyasa dynamic and incorporates invigorating, cleansing, and stimulating postures should be developed. A mandala in its basic form is a circle, which represents the spiraling upward motion that is encouraged in this sequence and echoes the mystical rising of kundalini shakti. It also symbolizes a cosmic diagram, based on the sacred geometry of the macrocosm as reflected in the microcosm of the human body. We use this sacred geometry in yoga to re-align the body in such a way that allows an even and balanced flow of energy. The Lotus Mandala Sequence contains many variations on *Padmasana*, the Lotus Pose, regarded as the ultimate posture for seated meditation, because while being stable, it is difficult to slump or collapse, thus encouraging a state of alertness. In Eastern art, the lotus flower, which grows on mud, represents purity and the tendency of the sublime essence to reveal itself only after an intense mental, emotional and physical engagement with life's challenges. What the yogi sets out to do is free themselves from this misidentification with conditioned existence and to still the fluctuating mind-states that result. The more adverse the

conditions that may be perceived to block us in our lives, as we enthusiastically and tenaciously tread the path of yoga, the more blissful the pink-white lotus blossom of the liberated state of consciousness will be.

Then you can embrace this existential mud as the very thing that roots and nourishes you, once you truly realize: you are not that.

The Lotus Mandala, as you can see in the image above, is used in Tibetan Buddhism (*Vajrayana*, the Tantric arm of Buddhism) as a visual aid for meditation. In its center is the *vajra*, which originally represented the diamond thunderbolt that cuts through ignorance, and also here in the Buddhist context symbolises the original crystalline purity. The Lotus Mandala Quantum Sequence starts and finishes in the Child's Pose and its Sublimatio consists of a *vajra-vinyasa* done on the toes. Not only does this fit into the symbolism of the mandala, it also necessitates a pulling up and away from gravity, engagement of the *bandhas*, and a hugging into your medial axis, all of which does not come naturally to the *kapha*-type. Yet, earth-water, once imbued with movement (pertaining to air) and the motivation to act (pertaining to fire) contains all the potential for conscious manifestation. Thus in the Lotus Mandala, the strength and stamina inherent in the human organism in particular and the universe as a whole is drawn upon to realign itself with its true sublime shape.

PRACTICING THE THREE BASIC QUANTUM SEQUENCES

Below you will find charts with illustrations, as well as lists of asana names. On the Quantum Yoga DVD contained in this book I demonstrate teaching each sequence to a yogi typical for their *dosha*-type. It is advisable that you watch these, before attempting to practice the sequence with the charts and lists below. To further facilitate the practice of the three Basic Quantum Sequences, double audio CDs of real-time instruction accompanied by beautiful music carefully selected to in turn ground, cool, and stimulate, are available on **www.quantumyoga.co.uk** or from selected outlets.

Note: Remember that whatever breath-count you choose, it must be even on both sides, unless you are consciously balancing a disharmony in your body. (See Chapter 3, *Timings*)

THE BIRDS SEQUENCE

The numbers besides the postures given below pertain to the numbering of the Birds chart photos.

SUBLIMATIO

(1) *Tadasana*: Feet together. Spread toes, engage *bandhas*, relax shoulders, lift sternum, open heart, begin *ujjai* breathing.

(2) Inhale, raise arms into *Urdhva Hastasana*.

(3) Exhale, hands down central line, move as if through water, feel energy of the life force like a prickling sensation in the palms of your hands.

(4) Inhale, arms up again. Interlock fingers and lift onto toes. Rotate to both sides on the out-breath, twisting from your core at the navel.

(5) & (6) Exhale, heels down to ground, change interlock of fingers, so opposite thumb is at the front. Inhale up again and exhale into the side-bends keeping feet evenly rooted.

DYNAMIC FLOW

(7)–(13): *Suryanamaskara*, Sun Salutation

Inhale, the arms rise for *Urdhva Hastasana* (2). Exhale, bend down into *Uttanasana* (8), inhale, look forward, spread the shoulders, and arch the spine *Ardha Uttanasana* (9). Exhale, bend your knees, place the palms firmly on the ground, and jump or step back into *Chaturanga Dandasana* (10). Inhale into *Urdhva Mukha Svanasana* (12), hold. Exhale, look over your

right shoulder (11), inhale center, exhale left, inhale center, exhale lift the sternum and pull the shoulders back more, inhale lift the gaze but keep the back of the neck long, exhale into:

(13) *Adho Mukha Svanasana*:

- shake head "yes" and "no" to release tension in neck
- spread palms and connect firmly to ground
- bend knees and stretch tailbone up or lift onto toes. Then release heels towards ground, while sustaining length and line of spine

Jump forward and inhale into *Ardha Uttanasana* (9). Exhale *Uttanasana* (8), inhale *Urdhva Hastasana* (7), *Exhale Samasthiti* (1).

Do another *Suryanamaskara* to *Adho Mukha Svanasana*.

(14) Step the right leg into Half-Pigeon and walk the hands forward. Be on the fingertips like the talons of a bird to create more space in the shoulders.

(15) Walk the hands back and place the right foot outside the hand in a lunge and bring the forearms to the floor if possible.

(16) Splits prep: Straighten the leg and lift the toes. Release the back leg heel down towards the ground.

Step back into *Adho Mukha Svanasana* (13) and repeat on the other side.

(17) From *Adho Mukha Svanasana*, walk the hands back to the

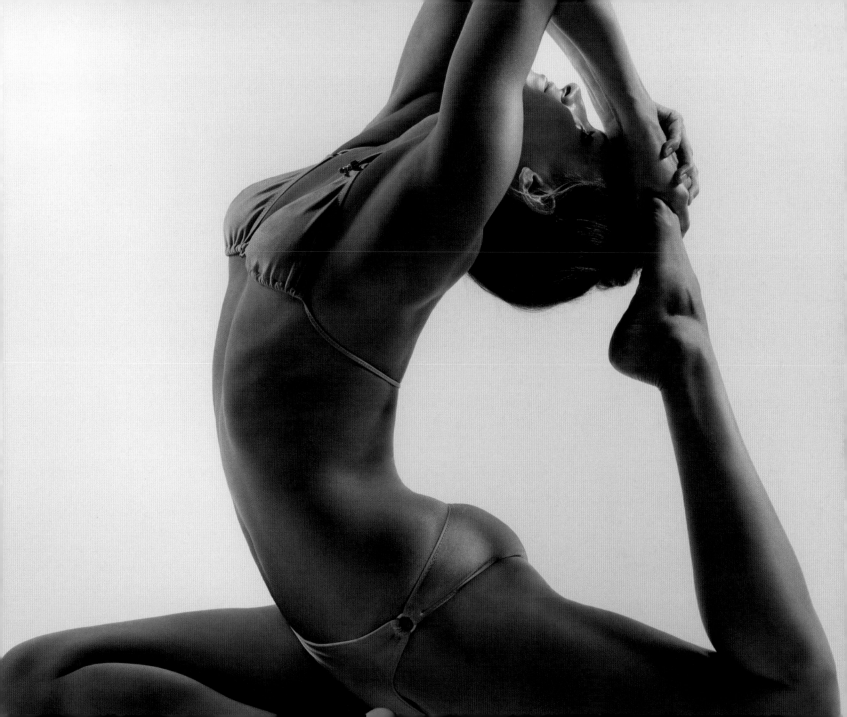

feet and hang forward, grabbing the elbows for *Uttanasana*. Pull the kneecaps up, grip the *bandhas*, breathe into the back and use gravity, releasing forward. Hold, and then leading with the elbows, inhale up, exhale and circumscribe a big circle with the tips of the fingers as you bring the hands to the hips.

(18) Turn the right heel in and step the left leg forward, bending the knee for *Virabhadrasana* 1 (Warrior 1). Inhale the arms up, palms together and *drishti* up.

(19) Now interlock the fingers, bar the index fingers. Bring your torso horizontal to the floor and lift the right leg off, while straightening the left leg. This is *Virabhadrasana* 3, the Warrior 3. Keep the pelvis level, the right foot toes pointing down, foot flexed, extending into the heel. Torso and right leg are parallel to the ground. Looking forward will give further lift and open the chest.

With control, lower the right foot down and come back into Warrior 1 **(18)**.

(20) From here we move into *Virabhadrasana* 2, the Warrior 2. Keeping the left leg bent, lower the arms down horizontally. Swing the right hip back, so the pelvis is flat. You may need to move your right foot a little further away and in line with the left. Looking to your right, draw the torso to center until it's perfectly vertical. Then look to your left, making sure the left knee is still above the heel, not collapsing inwards. Fix your gaze and sink even lower, drawing the navel back, tucking the tailbone under, lifting the sternum, but relaxing the shoulders.

Cartwheel the back arm over bringing the hands to the floor. From here do a half-*vinyasa*: exhale step back and lower to *Chatwari* **(10)**, inhale *Urdhva Mukha Svanasana* **(12)**, exhale to *Adho Mukha Svanasana* **(13)**.

(21) Walk your hands back to the feet. This time lift your feet and place the hands under so the palms are against the soles of your feet. Inhale, look forward, extend the spine, and broaden the shoulders. Exhale, release the head down into *Padahastasana*, Hand-to-Foot Pose.

Warriors 1, 3, 2 on other side and *vinyasa* to *Samastithi*.

(22) Inhale and sink into *Utkatasana*, bending your knees as though you were sitting down on an invisible chair, as you raise the arms up and direct your gaze to the outstretched fingertips.

Now lower yourself all the way down, spread your knees and bring your arms between the knees, resting the outer edge of your hands on the floor. Ideally the feet remain flat, but if the heels are lifting off the ground, you may want to use a block or fold up your mat beneath them for balance. Spread your back and once again draw the prana into the spine.

(23) If you want to try moving into the full *Malasana*, Garland Pose, wrap the arms around your bent legs, taking the armpits as close to the shins as possible. Now see whether you can catch your hands behind your back.

(24) Place your hands shoulder-width apart on the floor

in front of you for *Bakasana*, the Crow. Lift onto your toes and raise your knees, placing them onto the back of the arms, right up by the armpits. Now raise your bum, grip the *bandhas*, and allow the feet to lift off the floor. The eyes look straight ahead and the toes point back. Your back is arched like a dome, drawing the navel to the spine, the tailbone lifted. **(25)** From there, careful not to bang your toes, shoot the legs back and lower into *Chatwari*.

Half-*vinyasa* to *Adho Mukha Svanasana* **(13)**.

(26) Move into *Vasishtasana*, Pose of the Sage Vasishta: come onto the outer edge of your right foot and stack the left foot on top. Balance on the right arm and lift your left arm up towards the sky. Your body is at a diagonal; use the core stability from the *bandhas* to stop the hips from sagging down. Finally look up past your left hand, keeping *jalandhara bandha*, the chin drawn in, back of the neck long.

Do both sides with a half-*vinyasa* between.

STANDING POSES

Cross your hands in front of your heart and step out with your left leg about a leg-length apart, arms horizontal. Turn the right foot in slightly and the left foot out, so the heel of your left foot is in line with the instep of the right. Legs straight and gripped.

(27) Inhale, lift the sternum, exhale, lower your left hand to the left shin or floor, keeping the hips perfectly flat for

Trikonasana, the Triangle pose. Inhale, look up past your right hand, keeping the chin in and back of the neck long. Imagine your body on both sides flush against a wall. Open the sternum, raising the energy right into the tips of the fingers. Grip the legs and keep pulling your right hip up. Lengthen the torso horizontally from the tailbone right to the base of the skull.

(28) Now place the right hand onto the hipbone at the front, look down at your left foot, bend the knee and place the left hand about a foot in front of the foot, slightly on the pinkie-toe side. Then lift the right leg off the floor and straighten the standing leg for *Ardha Chandrasana*, the Half-Moon Pose. Raise the right hip, again coming two-dimensional and flat like in the Triangle. Once you have found balance, extend the right arm up vertical and look past the right hand. Come out the same way you went in, exhaling the right foot back the ground and inhaling into Triangle, exhale and inhale out of the pose. Swivel on your feet and then repeat the Triangle and Half-Moon on the other side.

Inhale up and swivel around squaring your hips up to the back. You may need to shorten and widen your stance somewhat, so that the right hip can swing around like in the Warrior 1. Now place your fingertips on the floor by either side of the left foot, leveling out the pelvis, extending the tailbone back and broadening the shoulders. Then shift the right hand to the left side of the left foot. If it doesn't reach the floor, place it on the shin or use a stable support under the hand for elevation.

(29) Keeping the hips level, extend the left arm up and look towards your left hand. This is *Parivrrita Trikonansana*, or the Revolving Triangle. Make sure the left shoulder is open and not scrunched up. Keep the back leg strong, pressing the foot down for support. Generate the twist from the spine itself, not by tilting the right hip down.

Leading with the right arm, on the inhalation come up. Exhale, swivel around on your feet, again adjusting their positioning so your hips are square to the front, legs straight.

Repeat on the other side and then step to *Samasthiti*. Then step out with the left leg again for the (30) *Parsvakonasana* variations. Draw the right foot in slightly and the left foot out, so that they are perpendicular and in line with each other. On the exhalation, bend the left knee to a right angle and place the left hand on the floor by the inner edge of the foot. Inhale, look up past your right hand, extending into the fingertips and opening the sternum.

(31) Bound *Parsvakonasana*: try bringing the left arm through the legs and catching the right hand or even the wrist behind your back. Then look up past the right shoulder and once again open the heart region.

Look down again and see how much you can straighten your left leg while keeping the bind. Then bend the knee again, slide the right foot in to the left heel and come onto the toes of your left foot, all the while keeping the arms bound (32).

(33) Now carefully on the inhalation without jerking lift the left leg off the floor and straighten the right. Broaden the sternum, draw the chin in and finally straighten your left leg too.

With control bring the left leg down again, knee bent at 90 degrees and step the right leg out.

(34) *Utthita Parsvakonasana*: release the bind and place the left hand on the floor by the outer edge of the left foot, stretch the right arm up on the inhale, rotate the arm forward, and exhale extend, forming a diagonal from right foot to right hand. Look up from underneath your armpit and then extend the gaze to the outstretched hand, keeping the back of your neck long, exercising your eyes.

Repeat other side

Inhale up and turn the feet so they are a leg-length apart and parallel to each with the toes slightly drawn in and the heels out. Hands on your hips.

(35) *Prasarita Padottanasana*: keep the belly drawn back and the tailbone tucked under as you inhale and look up to the sky, lifting the heart. Exhale, bend forward and place the hands, shoulder-with apart, between your feet. Inhale look forward again, coming right up to your fingertips to broaden the back and lengthen the spine and keeping that space, exhale forward, releasing the crown of the head down towards the floor.

(36) *Samakonasana*: walk the hands forward beneath the shoulders and begin walking the feet out to the sides. Keep the feet flat on the ground. Work to your own capacity, never forcing, and using the breath to relax into the pose.

(37) *Hanumanasana*: Now shorten the distance between the feet again and carefully walk the hands to either side of your left leg, swinging the right hip around. Lift the left foot toes up towards you and slide into the front splits, using the arms on the floor to control how far down you want to go. Practice gently and allow your body to release slowly into the pose using the breath and *bandhas* to protect from injury. Unless you're all the way down in the splits, the right knee should remain off the floor. Only when you can do so with square hips, do you release the right foot, pointing the toes back.

(38) *Paschimottanasana* in *Hanumanasana*: once you have come into the full pose safely, bring the torso into a forward bend. Shorten again and walk the hands to the other side, adjusting the feet as before. Lift the right foot toes and gently release down. Repeat.

Exhale step back and lower to *Chatwari* **(10)**, inhale *Urdhva Mukha Svanasana* **(12)**, exhale *Adho Mukha Svanasana* **(13)**, jump forward and inhale *Ardha Uttanasana* **(9)**, exhale *Uttanasana* **(8)**, inhale *Urdhva Hastasana* **(7)**, exhale *Samastithi* **(1)**.

STANDING BALANCES

Look down at your feet and check that they are together. Spread the toes. Focus your *drishti*, (viewpoint) on an immobile spot straight in front of you for balance. Grip the *bandhas*, deepen the breathing.

(39) *Vrikshasana*, Tree Pose: shift the weight gently over to the right foot, bringing the left leg up, so that the sole of the foot is against the inner thigh of the right leg and the left knee pointing to the left side. Make sure that the right hip doesn't swing along, but rather peel it open to the right, keeping the right foot flat and the leg straight. Now stretch the *namaste* hands up to the sky.

Then bring your arms down horizontal, bend your standing leg slightly and wrap the left leg around the right from the front, hooking the foot around at the back if you can. Cross the right arm over the left, then cross again and bring the palms together.

(40) *Garudasana*, the Eagle Pose: remaining as vertical as possible, as though you had a string coming out of your head attaching you to the ceiling, begin sinking down into a squat. Now slowly lift back up, keeping the balance and finally stretching the fingertips up to the sky, feeling the opening in the shoulders and upper back. Release the arms and finally the legs.

Repeat on the other side.

FLOOR WORK

(This mini-sequence is done all on one side and then in reverse order on the opposite side as below:)

Do a full *vinyasa* to *Adho Mukha Svanasana*.

(41) Step your left leg once again into the One-Legged Pigeon Pose, *Eka Pada Kapotasana*, so that the left heel is just below the right hipbone. Again if you need to, use a small prop to elevate the left hip. This time walk your hands in to the sides of your hip, drawing in from your core at the navel and gripping the perineum. Look up to the sky, lifting the heart, dropping the shoulders.

(42) Look forward again, and placing your left hand by the knee, look over your right shoulder towards your back leg, bend the right knee and catch the instep of the right foot with your free hand. For most people this is a sufficiently strong stretch, but if you would like to move into a variation of the king pigeon, *Raja Kapotasana*, then slide the right foot into the right elbow, bring the left arm up behind your head and catch the hands in a monkey-grip, looking up past your left elbow. Avoid collapsing over to the left, by bringing the weight into your right hip.

(43) Release out of the pose and swing the right leg over to the front, pulling the left knee slightly to the left, so the legs end up in a right angle for *Janu Sirsasana*, Head-To-Knee Pose. Place the right hand on the floor by the side of the hip, stretch the left arm up, lengthening the spine and then grab the outer edge of the right foot or shin and look over your right shoulder, opening the sternum, involving the whole spine in the twist. Now look to your right foot and grab it with both hands, laying your spine along the leg. If you cannot reach the foot, use a belt, always wrapping it around the broadest part of the foot. Use the breath coupled with the *bandhas* to go deeper into this forward bend.

Inhale, the arms rise, exhale release them down to your side.

(44) Moving into *Ardha Matsyendrasana* now, bend your right leg slightly and slide your left foot over to the right side of the hip, so that the left knee is pointing straight forward. Then place the right foot down by the left side of the left knee. Place the right hand on the ground behind you, extend the left arm up, stretching the spine, then bend the elbow and stemming it against the right knee, look over your right shoulder and twist. Every time you inhale lengthen the spine, every time you exhale twist a little deeper. If you would like to try going into the full pose, then stemming your left shoulder against the knee, try to grab the right foot. Then swing the right arm around the back, grasping the left upper thigh with your right hand. Make sure to keep your foundation, both buttocks on the floor.

(45) Release out of the twist and now simply slide your right foot to the left side of the left hip, stacking the knees on top of each other for *Gomukhasana*, Cow's Head Pose. If you

are unstable, stick a pillow or block beneath your sitting bones. Now stretch the arms out to the side, rotate the right shoulder forward and bring the arm under, rotate the left shoulder back and bring the arm over, catching the hands in a monkey grip behind the back. If you can't catch, use a belt, or just reach as best as you can. Inhale, look up to the sky, and keeping the left elbow lifted, extend forward, again grounding the sitting bones as you bend forward. Breathe into the tight areas, creating space and releasing stress and blockages from the body. Inhale up, free the hands.

To change sides, you can leave the feet where they are, lean forward, lifting the bum off to do a 360-degree spin around turn to the left and sit back down between your feet. You should be in *Gomukhasana* again, this time with the left leg above the right.

(45) *Gomukhasana* on the opposite side

(44) *Ardha Matsyendrasana* to **(43)** *Janu Sirsasana*

Swing left leg back to **(41)** do Half-Pigeon with right leg, torso vertical looking up, then **(42)** *Eka Pada Raja Kapotasana* variation.

Place hands to ground, tuck back foot toes under and step back into *Adho Mukha Svanasana* **(13)**, inhale to Plank Pose, exhale to *Chatwari*, and lie down on belly.

BACKBENDS

(46) *Shalabhasana* x 2: lie down on your belly for the Locust, (*Shalabhasana*). The legs are together as you interlock the fingers behind your back. On the next exhalation, lift the arms, chest and legs off the ground and breathe. Keep lifting up, even getting those upper thighs off the ground. Stretch back into the toes and open the heart, looking up or straight ahead to keep the neck free.

Release.

Take the arms forward and interlock the fingers the opposite way and place the palms against the back of your head. If your legs have moved apart, bring them back together. Now once again lift into *Shalabhasana*, this time extending the elbows up, pressing the head against the hands. Lift and breathe. Release and push yourself back into pose of the child, *Balasana*, bending the knees, bum resting on the heels. Come to kneeling with knees and feet in line and hip-width apart.

(47) *Ushtrasana*: inhale, raise the arms, exhale, bring the hands in *namaste* in front of your heart and start leaning back, working the upper thighs and tightening the grip at the perineum. Eventually lower yourself into the Camel Pose, bringing the hands ideally together and at the same time to the heels. If you cannot reach, tuck your toes under. Finally relax the head back. Do not give your weight to the hands; they are simply here to encourage the opening of the thoracic region and chest. Instead drop the tailbone and move the pubic bone forward. Breathe deep and steady, calming the mind.

Rest in *Balasana* and repeat.

Sit up, place the hands beside knees, lift the body off floor, cross the legs, and swing through to sitting. Place soles of feet together for **(48)** *Baddha Konasana*, Bound Angle Pose. Wrap the hands around your feet. Inhale, fill the ribcage, exhale, extend forward, lowering your head towards the floor, but always leaving the sitting bones glued to the ground. Allow the knees to relax down, breathing into the hips, drawing the shoulders back and wide.

(*Optional Peak Pose*): torso upright, slide one leg back for Pigeon **(41)** and take yourself into full **(49)** *Eka Pada Raja Kapotasana*, the one-legged King Pigeon. Use a block under the Pigeon Leg bum for stability and a belt around the back foot, so you can walk the hands slowly towards the foot while learning this pose. Eventually once the hips and shoulders are sufficiently open and this deep backbend is possible, you can dispense with the props. Strong engagement of the *bandhas* is crucial here to sustain balance and protect the lower back! Do both sides. **(50)** *Upavishta Konasana*: inhale up, release your feet, and extend your legs out to the front, spreading them at a right angle for the Seated Angle Pose. Engage the legs, making sure that both knees and toes are pointing up. Now inhale, fill the heart, exhale bend forward, sliding the hands along the legs, reaching for the feet and ultimately wrapping index and middle fingers around the big toes. Make sure not to hunch your back, nor should you tilt your pelvis forward if you are very flexible.

ABDOMINALS

(51) *Upavishta Konasana*: sitting up, lift the legs off the floor, wrapping index and middle fingers around the big toes again. If you can't catch, either bend your knees or grab your shins instead. Reinforce *mula bandha* for balance. Look forward and slightly up to encourage the lift of the sternum. Pull the shoulder blades out and down.

Move the legs together and lift the *drishti* for **(52)** *Ubhaya Padanghustasana*.

Release the toes and bring the hands to the side of the legs, palms facing each other.

(53) *Navasana*, the Boat Pose. Make sure not to collapse the spine; bend the knees if you have to. Again lift the heart and draw the thoracic spine in. Lie down for the dynamic *Navasana* (exhale up, hold empty, inhale down) leading the smooth movement with the head, then arms, torso, and legs with *mula* and *uddhiyana bandha* on *bhaya kumbhaka*. Do at least five repetitions.

INVERSIONS

(Moon-day girls relax in *Supta Baddha Konasana* with belt and bolster and from there to *Savasana*.)

(54) *Halasana*: bring your legs carefully over and back now, slowly lowering the toes to the ground for the *Plow*. Be very mindful of your neck and keep your gaze throughout this sequence glued to the belly button. If it's too much, just roll out! Interlock your fingers behind the back, and carefully wiggle further onto the tops of your shoulders. Legs are straight. Lift your tailbone up towards the sky, lengthening the spine.

(55) *Salamba Sarvangasana*: support your back with your hands and carefully lift your legs into the Shoulderstand. Engage the legs, extending into the whole sole of the foot, as though you wanted to stand on the sky. You may want to spread the legs a little and tuck the tailbone under, before bringing them back together. Carefully walk the hands further towards your shoulder blades, thereby increasing the verticality of the pose. Now slow down and deepen the breath!

If you feel confident here, you may want to try the unsupported Shoulderstand, *Niralamba Sarvangasana*, by extending the arms up by the side of your body. If this is too difficult, you could also try laying the arms down by the side of the head. Grip the *bandhas* for balance and lift!

(56) *Karnapidasana*: now slowly lower the legs back down. Bend the knees, bringing them to the side of the ears and wrap the arms around the legs, curling up into the Ear-Pressure Pose.

Slowly, vertebra by vertebra, massaging your spine, roll out of the pose.

(57) *Matsyasana*: now push into the elbows and lift the torso off the floor for the Fish pose. Hang your head back and carefully lower the crown of the head down to the ground. Draw the thoracic spine in and open the heart. Staying there, lift the arms up and bring the hands into prayer, stretching them in the direction of your gaze. Fingers and toes pointing in opposing directions.

Bring the arms over again, push into the elbows, lift the chin to the sternum and gently lower the head down.

(58) *Pavanmuktasana*, neck twists: bend your knees and wrap your arms around the knees, lifting the head off the floor. Look to your right, center, then the left, center, and release the head down again.

(59) *Savasana*, the Corpse Pose: look up at your feet to check that your body is in a straight line. Then lay your arms by the side of your torso, palms facing up. Some people like to place an eye-bag or a rolled-up cloth over their eyes in Savasana. Relax! Be happy and free.

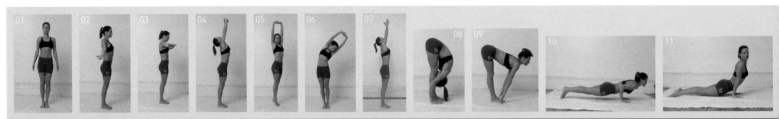

01 TADASANA: MOUNTAIN POSE 02 ARMS RISE 03 PALMS DOWN CENTRE 04 LIFT TO TOES 05 ROTATE ON TOES 06 STANDING SIDE BEND 07 URDHVA HASTASANA: UPWARD EXTENDED ARMS
08 UTTANASANA: STANDING FORWARD BEND 09 ARDHA UTTANASANA: HALF FORWARD BEND 10 CHATURANGA DANDASANA (CHATWARI): PRESS-UP 11 UP-DOG HEAD TURNED

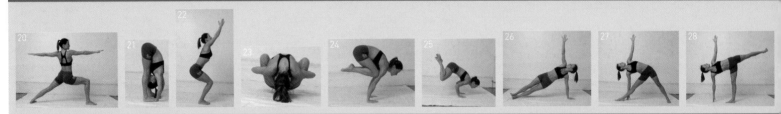

20 VIRABHADRASANA 2: WARRIOR 2 21 PADA HASTASANA: HAND TO FOOT POSE 22 UTKATASANA: AWKWARD POSE 23 MALASANA: GARLAND 24 BAKASANA: CROW 25 JUMP BACK TO PRESS-UP
26 VASISHTASANA: SAGE VASISHTA 27 UTTHITA TRIKONASANA: EXTENDED TRIANGLE 28 ARDHA CHANDRASANA: HALF-MOON

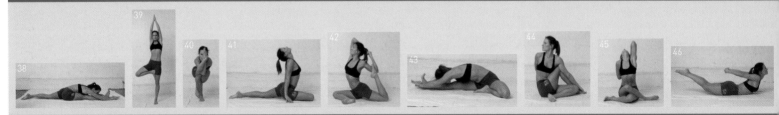

39 VRIKSHASANA: TREE 40 GARUDASANA: EAGLE 41 EKA PADA KAPOTASANA: ONE-LEGGED PIGEON 42 EKA PADA RAJA KAPOTASANA: ONE-LEGGED KING PIGEON
43 JANU SHIRSASANA: HEAD TO KNEE 44 ARDHA MATSUYENDRASANA: HALF LORD OF THE FISH 45 GOMUKHASANA: HEAD OF COW 46 SHALABHASANA: LOCUST

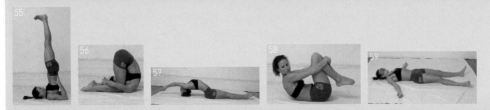

55 SALAMBA SARVANGASANA: SUPPORTED SHOULDER-STAND 56 KARNAPIDASANA: EAR-PRESSURE 57 MATSUYASANA: FISH 58 PAVANMUKTASANA 59 SHAVASANA: CORPSE

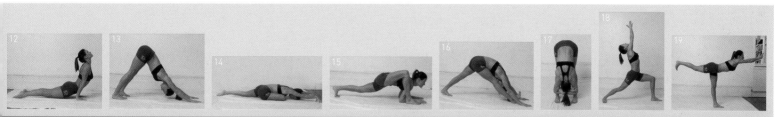

12 URDHVA MUKHA SVANASANA: UPWARD-FACING DOG **13** ADHO MUKHA SVANASANA: DOWNWARD-FACING DOG **14** EKA PADA KAPOTASANA: ONE-LEGGED PIGEON **15** LIZARD LUNGE **16** SPLITS PREPARATION **17** UTTANASANA: STANDING FORWARD BEND **18** VIRABHADRASANA 1: WARRIOR 1 **19** VIRABHADRASANA 3: WARRIOR 3

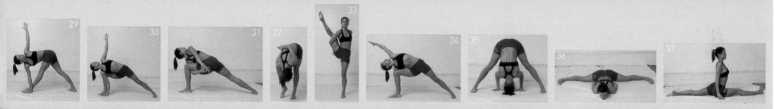

29 PARIVRITTA TRIKONASANA: REVOLVING TRIANGLE **30, 31, 32, 33, 34** UTTHITA PARSVAKONASA: EXTENDED LATERAL ANGLE VARIATIONS **35** PRASARITA PADOTTANSANA: INTENSE SPREAD LEG STRETCH **36** SAMAKONASA: GREAT ANGLE **37 & 38** HANUMANASA: MONKEY

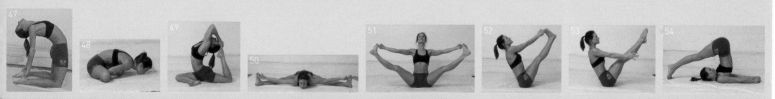

47 USHTRASANA: CAMEL **48** BADHA KONASANA: BOUND ANGLE **49** EKA PADA RAJA KAPOTASANA: ONE-LEGGED KING PIGEON **50 & 51** UPAVISHTA KONASANA: SEATED ANGLE **52** UBHAYA PADANGHUSTASANA: THUMBS TO FEET **53** NAVASANA: BOAT **54** HALASANA: PLOW

THE HEROES SEQUENCE

The numbers besides the postures given below pertain to the numbering of the Heroes chart photos.

PRANAYAMA

(1) *Supta Baddha Konasana* with props
Viloma Pranayama (three-part inhalation with *antara kumbhaka* from bottom to top of body; should not be done by persons who suffer from hypertension, hernia or any other lesions to the abdominal wall).

SUBLIMATIO

(2) Squat with feet together and soles flat on floor and knees squeezing together. Support heels with block if necessary. Stretch arms, hands in prayer, up to the sky. Be as upright as possible!
(3) Lift tailbone, wrap forearms around calves and come into *Uttanasana* with torso in contact with thighs (knees bent if necessary).
(4) Release, hang arms forward, straighten legs, and from there unfold vertebra by vertebra.
(5) From *Tadasana*, Mountain Pose, step out for
(6) *Ashvarohinasana* (Horse-Riding Stance).
Place hands in *Namaste* in front of heart (*anjali* mudra). Chant each *bija* mantra three times and visualize the chakra in question (you can use color, contemplate spiritual significance, or psychological or developmental condition related to the chakra).

• *LAM: Muladhara* (root) chakra. Color: red.
• *VAM: Swadisthana* (between pubic bone and navel) chakra. Color: orange.
• *RAM: Manipura* (solar plexus) Chakra. Color: yellow.
  - Rest -
• *YAM: Anahata* (heart center) chakra. Color: green.
• *HAM: Vissudhi* (throat) chakra. Color: blue.
• *AUM: Ajna* ("third" eye) chakra. Color: violet.
  - Rest -
• Repeat all one time.
• Hold *silence*, hear the resonance of *aum* and visualize *sahasrara* (crown) chakra as a transparent halo of light or a thousand-petaled multicolored lotus floating above the head, beyond the physical confines of the body.
Scoop arms down, straighten legs, and step into *Samasthiti*.

FLOWING STANDING SEQUENCE

(7)–(14) *Suryanamaskara* A with three full breaths in *Urdhva Mukha Svanasana* looking over left shoulder, right, center, up. Several breaths in *Adho Mukha Svanasana*, back to (7) *Samasthiti*. Full vinyasa to *Adho Mukha Svanasana*. Step one leg forward, heel in line with instep, straighten legs as you unfold into (15) *Trikonasana*, hold for three to six breaths. Extended hand down. Step back foot somewhat shorter and wider, pull heel back, and if necessary place brick under supporting hand and unfold into (16) *Parivritta Trikonasana*, hold for three to six breaths

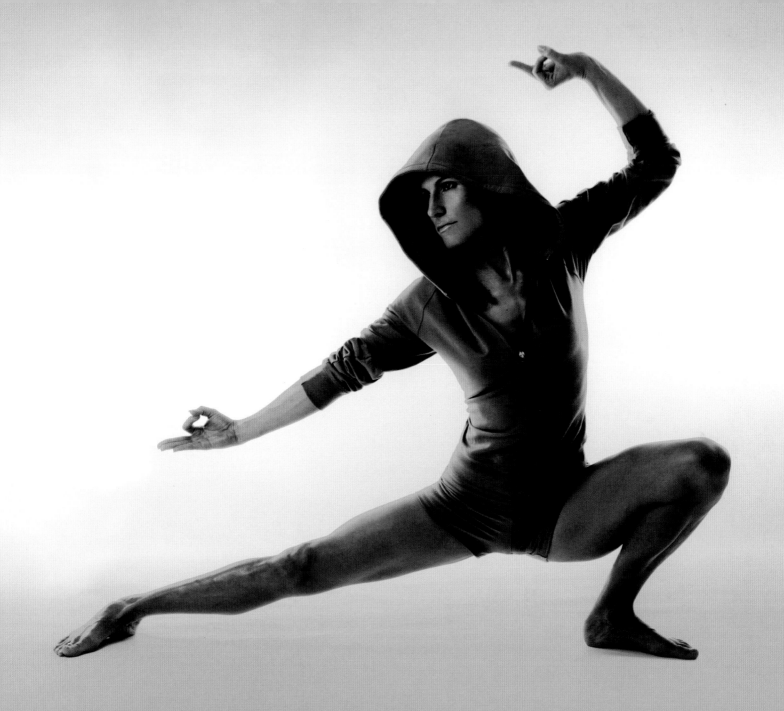

Exhale, hand down, inhale, look forward, bend front leg knee and tuck back foot toes under, exhale swing the leg back and up into **(17)** *Eka Pada Svanasana* (One-Legged Dog)
inhale forward into Three-Legged Plank, exhale lower to *Chatwari*, from here normal half-*vinyasa* to *Adho Mukha Svanasana*. Repeat Triangle and Rotated Triangle on the other side.

Do the same half-*vinyasa* variation as before. (Full *vinyasa* to *Samasthiti* is also good here to demarcate the new set of standing poses). From *Adho Mukha Svanasana* step one leg forward for **(18)** *Utthita Parsvakonasana*.

From there bring the extended hand down. If necessary, step back foot somewhat shorter and wider and pull heel back. Place opposing elbow against outer bent leg knee and twist into **(19)** or **(20)** *Parivritta Parsvakonasana*.

Half-*vinyasa* variation to *Adho Mukha Svanasana*. Repeat Lateral Angle Pose and Rotated Lateral Angle Pose on the other side.

Full *vinyasa* to *Samasthiti*. Step out for **(21)** Horse-Riding Stance. Hands in *jnana* mudra (index and thumb fingertips touching. Arms crossed in front of the chest).

(22) and **(23)** The Archer, *Dhanushmatasana*
Begin with arm movements, one palm face-up overhead, the other reaching out.

Then bring in leg movement, arm still horizontal.

Then dip low and "shoot arrow" into the ground by the foot, so the arm is at a diagonal with the leg. Feet must remain grounded. Torso as upright as possible, chest lifted.

Finally, try inhaling into the Archer and exhaling to center in Horse **(21)**, inhaling into the Archer on the other side, thus keeping the center of gravity low throughout. Sustain the *vinyasa*-flow by moving continuously with the breath.

To center into Horse and turn feet in, straighten legs. Hands to hips. Inhale, look up and lift the heart space, exhale into **(24)** *Prasarita Padottanasana*. Inhale up again.

Come to kneeling on one leg, with the hip stacked exactly above it. Place the heel of the other leg, which should be straight, in line with the opposing bent knee. Make sure the foot is flat on the ground.

(25) Inhale the arms up, as though embracing an egg of energy, exhale, side-bend into **(26)** *Parighasana* with one arm sliding down the extended leg, keep the bent-leg hip above the knee.

Sweep through to horizontal arms and set up for the other side.

When you've done the Gate Pose on both sides, sweep the other arm through to horizontal and come to kneeling.

(27)–**(33)** Quantum Mini-Sequence
Place the hands shoulder-width apart on the mat and the head in front of the hands, so that if you drew a line between the three points of contact, the shape would be that of a triangle. Keep the elbows above the wrists, as you walk the pelvis over the shoulder-girdle and float or hop up into three-point *Shirsanana* **(27)**. From thereon the exhalation

move the knees as high up onto the forearms as possible **(28)** and pushing strongly through the arms, inhale lift the head off the ground to look forward for *Bakasana* **(29)**, the Crow. Exhale the head back down and ride the momentum as you straighten the legs back up into *Shirsasana*. Inhale, point the toes and spread the legs **(30)**. When you can't go any further, exhale, flex the feet **(31)**, tilt the pelvis and lower the legs **(32)** to *Prasarita Padottanasana* **(24)**. As soon as the feet touch the floor, inhale look forward, and spread the sternum **(33)**, exhale hands to hips, inhale grip the bandhas as you lift up, exhale step back to *Samastithi*. (Safety note: should you fall from three-point headstand the most important thing is to pull the chin in and allow the body to roll out. Therefore make sure there are no sharp objects or other yogis in the way.)

STANDING BALANCES

Hands to hips, bend knees, fix drishti for the **(34)**–**(36)** *Shiva Natarajasana*, *Dancing Shiva* variations.
Keeping the standing leg knee bent, lift the other leg up and point the toes to the opposing side. Straighten the arms ahead of you and place the hands on top of each other. Bend the wrists, so fingertips are pointing up and down **(34)**.
Grab the energy in the palms of your hands and hold the cupped hands in front of your *kanda* (core, just below the navel). Straighten both legs and extend into the ball of the foot **(35)**.
Bend the extended leg and bring the knees together, while

pointing the toes back. Take the hand out like you are asking someone to dance and grab the instep of that foot. Place the straight leg hand in *jnana* mudra and reach forward. Unfold into *Shiva Natarajasana* **(36)**, pointing the bent leg toes to the sky, while the knee points down to keep the hips level. Lift the chest.
Release back into *Tadasana* and repeat all three Dancing Shiva variations on the other side.

FLOOR WORK

Do a *vinyasa* to *Adho Mukha Svanasana*. To learn how to jump into the next pose **(37)**, you could practice by bending ideally first the left knee to the face, while dragging the foot along the floor, and then bringing the right leg through **(38)**. Inhale the arms up and exhale forward into
(39) *Triangmukaekapada Paschimottanasana*
• Place a block under the straight leg buttock if necessary and keep the knees together.
Inhale up from there. Hug the right leg into the body, grab the foot (use a belt if necessary), and come into
(40) and **(41)** *Kraunchasana*, looking up first to lift the chest and flatten the thoracic spine **(40)** and then exhaling the face to the leg **(41)**.
(42) and **(43)** *Bharadvajasana*
• Place the right leg into the Half-Lotus. You can spread the legs a little now.
• If necessary, support the Lotus knee or even straighten out

the Hero's leg.

• Place the right hand behind you (on a block if necessary), the left hand on the right Lotus knee and twist to the right **(42)**.

• If you can go into the full posture, bind the right index and middle finger around the Lotus big toe. Place the left hand under the right knee with the palm facing down and twist to the right in this manner **(43)**. Keep the left sitting-bone grounded.

Undo the legs. Do a half *vinyasa* and repeat the Heroes Floor Sequence on the other side.

Do a half *vinyasa*. From *Adho Mukha Svanasana*, come into *Balasana* with the arms stretched forward, hands shoulder-width apart **(44)**.

BACKBENDS

(44)–(46) Child–Cobra Sequence

From *Balasana*, inhale onto all fours, exhale, lower the body down, inhale lift into *Bhujangasana* **(45)**. Exhale the chest down, and leading with the sitting-bones, bring the bum back to the heels **(46)**. Repeat three to six times, synchronizing breath and movement in a flow. On the last one hold the Cobra **(45)** for three breaths and then lie flat for

(47) *Ardha-Bhekasana*

• They may spread a little, but always initiate the Frog with the legs together. Place one arm perpendicular to the body, beneath the chest to prop the torso up. Look over the opposite shoulder, bend that knee and grab the instep of the foot with your free hand. Lift the elbow, pivot the wrist and press down on the foot, so that the fingers are draped over and pointing in the same direction as the toes, and the palm is asserting even pressure on the foot. Repeat on the opposite side. Then try the full Frog:

(48) *Bhekasana*

Grab both insteps. Inhale the torso off the floor, pivot both wrists, positioning the hands to exhale and press the feet down.

Do a half *vinyasa* or simply turn onto your back for the **(49)–(51)** Moving *Urdhva Dhanurasana* (like upside-down press-ups). Place the hands palms down beneath the shoulders. Stack the elbows above the wrists. Bend the knees and place the feet hip-width and parallel to each other, stacking the knees above the heels **(49)**. Exhale, lift onto the crown of the head **(50)**. Inhale, consolidate your foundation, palms and soles flat on the ground. Exhale lift up. Inhale look to the sky and increase the heart-opening **(51)**. Keep that breadth as you exhale and relax your head into *Urdhva Dhanurasana* **(51)**. Inhale back onto the crown of your head. Exhale, pull the elbows in and the heels out. Inhale back up. Exhale look to the sky, push carefully through the legs. Inhale relax the head, exhale back to the crown. Synchronizing alternating breath counts with the movement, continue the flow, eventually working up to six backbends.

COUNTERPOSE & CORE

(53) Cradle

Place the feet together, wrap the clasped hands around the shins, tuck the tailbone under and lean back, reinforcing *mula* and *uddhiyana bandha*.

(54) Cosmic Egg

Move the legs in closer, wrap the arms around the legs, catching the elbows with the hands and float the feet off the floor. Close the eyes and enjoy the feeling of weightlessness. Keep the breath powerful but soften its quality.

INVERSIONS

(55)–(57) *Sarvangasana* with alternate leg-raisers

(Moon-day girls go into *Supa Baddha Konasana* **(1)** or skip to **(61)** for the couch and **(62)** the Supine Hero's Pose.)

Take the legs over into *Halasana* **(55)**, interlock the fingers behind the back, lift onto the shoulders, careful to protect the neck. Support the back with the hands and lift into *Salamba Sarvangasana* **(56)**. Exhale one leg down, inhale it back up again. Alternate. Attention is with the static leg, which remains totally vertical and does not turn out. Cultivate pelvic integrity. **(57)**

Keep the back supported by the hands, as you lower the legs back into Plow and then spread them to a right angle for

(58) *Supta Konasana*.

(59) *Parsva Karnapidasana*

Walk one leg to the other. Bend the knees and take them to the side of the head, opposite arm flat on the ground as a counterweight.

Straighten legs, replace hand against back and legs to *Supta Konasana* **(58)** again.

Repeat on the opposite side.

Narrow the angle of the legs, bend the knees and wrap them around the ears for

(60) *Karnapidasana*.

Roll out.

RELAXATION

Sit up, cross the legs, roll onto the knees, and tuck the legs under. Knees together and feet hip-width apart, lower the sitting bones to the floor. If the bum doesn't reach the floor, use a block for support and set up a bolster behind you.

(61) *Paryankasana*

Lean back on your elbows, lower the crown of the head to the floor, grab the elbows and bring them overhead. Hold for a few breaths and then lower into

(62) *Supta Virasana*.

To come out, pull up the knees one by one and then slide the feet away or sit up, undo the legs and then lie back in

(63) *Savasana*.

Close your eyes and surrender all action, thoughts or even dreams, and instead just be!

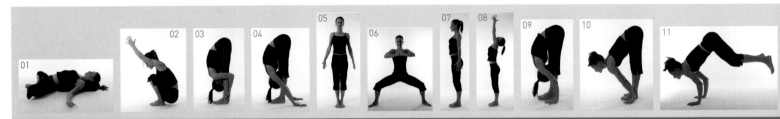

01 SUPTA BADHA KONASANA: SUPINE BOUND ANGLE 02 UTKATASANA: AWKWARD POSE 03, 04 UTTANASANA: STANDING FORWARD BEND 05 TADASANA: MOUNTAIN 06 HORSE-RIDING STANCE
07 TADASANA: MOUNTAIN 08 URDVHA HASTASANA: UPWARD EXTENDED ARMS 09 UTTANASANA: STANDING FORWARD BEND 10 ARDHA UTTANSANA: HALF STANDING FORWARD BEND
11 JUMP BACK

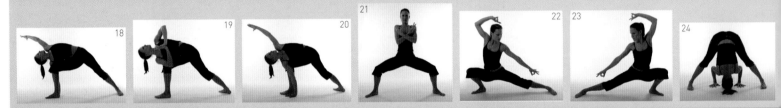

18 UTTHITA PARSVAKONASANA: EXTENDED LATERAL ANGLE POSE 19 & 20 PARIVRTTA PARSVAKONASANA: ROTATED LATERAL ANGLE POSE
21 JNYANA MUDRA IN ASHVAROHINASANA: SEAL OF WISDOM IN HORSE 22 & 23 DHANUSHMATASANA: ARCHER 24 PRASARITA PADOTTANASANA: INTENSE SPREAD LEG STRETCH

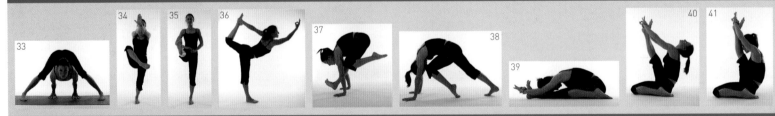

33 ARDHA PADOTTANASANA: HALF SPREAD LEG STRETCH 34, 35 & 36 SHIVANATARAJASANA: DANCING SHIVA 37 VINYASA JUMP 38 VINYASA ALTERNATIVE
39 TRIANGMUKAEKAPADA PASCHIMOTTANASANA: THREE-POINT FORWARD BEND 40 & 41 KROUNCHASANA: HERON

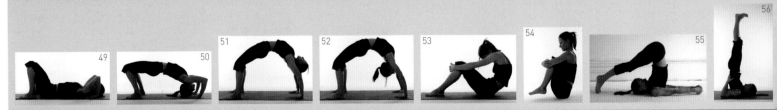

49 & 50 URVHA Dhanurasana INTRO 51 & 52 URDVHA Dhanurasana: UPWARD BOW 53 CRADLE 54 BRAHMANDASANA: COSMIC EGG 55 HALASANA: PLOUGH
56 SALAMBA SARVANGASANA: SUPPORTED SHOULDERSTAND

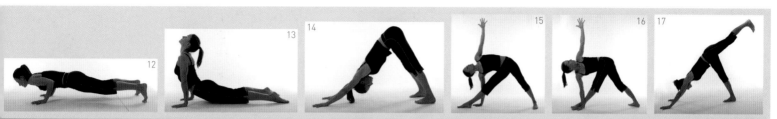

12 CHATURANGA DANDASANA (CHATWARI): PRESS-UP POSE 13 URDHVA MUKHA SVANASANA: UPWARD-FACING DOG 14 ADHO MUKHA SVANASANA: DOWNWARD-FACING DOG
15 UTTHITA TRIKONASANA: EXTENDED TRIANGLE 16 PARIVRTTA TRIKONASANA: ROTATED TRIANGLE 17 EKA PADA SVANASANA: ONE-LEGGED DOG

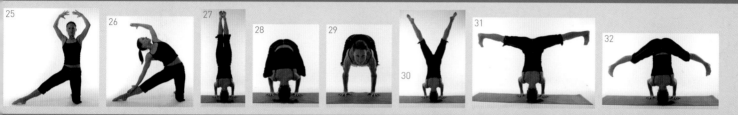

25 PARIGHASANA PRELUDE 26 PARIGHASANA: GATE 27 SHIRSASANA: HEADSTAND 28 BAKASANA PRELUDE 29 BAKASANA: CROW 30, 31 & 32 SHIRSASANA DESCENT

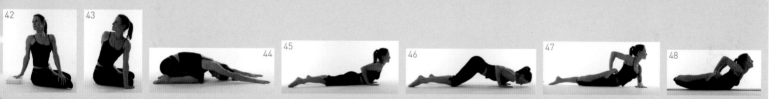

42 & 43 BHARADVAJASANA: SAGE BHARADVAJA 44 BALASANA: CHILD 45 BHUJANGHASANA: COBRA 46 COBRA-CHILD TRANSITION 47 ARDHA BEKASANA: HALF FROG 48 BEKASANA: FROG

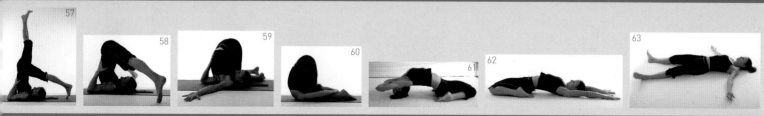

57 EKA PADA SARVANGASANA: ONE-LEGGED SHOULDERSTAND 58 SUPTA KONASANA: SUPINE ANGLE POSE 59 PARSVA KARNAPIDASANA: SIDE EAR-PRESSURE POSE
60 KARNAPIDASANA: EAR-PRESSURE POSE 61 PARYANKASANA: COUCH 62 SUPTA VIRASANA: SUPINE HERO 63 SHAVASANA: CORPSE

THE LOTUS MANDALA SEQUENCE

The numbers besides the postures given below pertain to the numbering of the Lotus Mandala chart photos.

SUBLIMATIO

(1) and (2) *Balasana* with kidney breathing
Alternate anus/genital plexus sqeeze, to prepare for the isolation of *mula bandha*, engagement of the perineum, and lifting of the pelvic floor.
(3) Sit up, separate knees, and place hands on the floor. Stick your tongue out and exhale in Lion Breath to empty. Hold the breath out, close your mouth, and draw the navel back and up: *uddhiyana bandha* on *bhaya kumbhaka*.

INTRO

Vajra-Vinyasas
(4) Draw the knees together, place the hands on the floor and roll over the toes, backwards and forwards.
(5) Be on the tops of the feet, interlock the fingers, rotate the wrists and stretch from the elbows into the palms. Scoop the tailbone under, drawing the navel back, and float the knees off the floor. Release back down.
Tuck the toes under, sit on the heels, lift the arms in the same manner, alternating the interlock of the fingers, so that the opposite thumb is on the top. Carefully draw the knees up off the floor (do not yank! If you need to push yourself off with the hands, please do.)
(6) *Vajrasana*
Inhale up to standing, still on your toes.

(7) Exhale twist to your side, rotating from the core at your navel. Squeeze knees and ankles together for balance. Inhale to center. Exhale to the other side. Inhale to center. Exhale hands and heels down.
(8) *Tadasana*
Interlock the hands the opposite way, so that the other thumb is on top. Inhale them back up your center and lift onto the toes.
Exhale and bend to the side. Inhale to center. Exhale to the other side. Inhale to center.
Exhale into *Vajrasana* (6) and lower the knees carefully to the floor.
(9) Place the clasped hands on the ground, but keep the sitting bones in contact with the heels. Do *bandha triyam* on *bhaya kumbhaka* (reinforcing all three *bandhas* on empty).
(10) Inhale the arms back up again and exhale, place the palms on the ground behind you, lifting the sitting bones off the heels.
Inhale the arms back up again and exhale take the hands in *namaste* down your center, placing them on the ground and lifting into
(11) *Vajra-Uttanasana*
Lower the sitting bones again for *Vajrasana* (6) and twist to both sides, keeping the knees together and level.
Exhale the knees down, release the toes and come onto all fours.

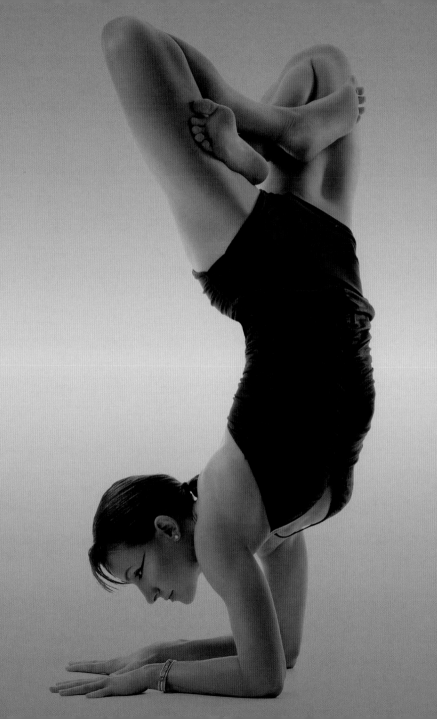

(12) and (13) Cat

Inhale, look up, and concave the spine (14). Draw the shoulder blades down and stretch the tailbone to the sky.

Exhale, look down, and convex the spine, reinforcing the *bandhas* on empty.

Repeat several times, involving every single vertebra in the movement.

(14) Still on all fours for the pelvic stability exercise, inhale opposing leg and arm up to horizontal. Keep the spine neutral and the sacrum level. Flexing the foot and extending into the heel will help. Hold for three breaths.

Exhale the limbs back down and inhale the other opposing pair up. Hold for three breaths.

Now do the same in a continuous *vinyasa*-flow, inhaling alternate leg and arm up, and exhaling down again. Once you have done an even amount of times on both sides, tuck the toes under and come into

(15) *Adho Mukha Svanasana*

(16) *Eka Pada Svanasana*

Lift one leg to horizontal, flexing the foot and extending into the heel. Keep the sacrum level!

(17) *Eka Pada Svanasana* Twist

Now lift the same leg up and over, bend the knee, and point the toes to the opposing side. Hips are now stacked on top of each other. Keep the head hanging down and hit the outer thigh of the standing leg back strongly. Keep the weight distribution on the hands even.

Exhale the leg back to horizontal, leveling the sacrum (16) and then place the foot down for *Adho Mukha Svanasana* (15).

Rest in the Child's Pose (1) and (2) if necessary. Repeat the One-Legged Dog variations on the opposite side.

In *Adho Mukha Svanasana* (15), blubber your lips a few times, before you jump forward into *Samasthiti* (8).

Step the feet to edge of mat and swing the arms around, rotating from the hips.

(18) Jump your feet together and jump up and down with the arms moving freely.

Come back into *Tadasana* (8) with the eyes closed. Allow all the microscopic particles of energy to settle, finding a new and better distribution. Slow down your breath and let the central alignment of the *bandhas* grow from the inside out in your endeavor to cultivate all the qualities of a mountain.

DYNAMIC FLOW

(19)–(28) Lotus Mandala *Suryanamaskara*

Inhale, the arms rise for *Urdhva Hastasana* (19). Exhale bend down into *Uttanasana* (20), inhale, look forward, spread the shoulders and arch the spine *Ardha Uttanasana* (21). Bend your knees, place the palms firmly on the ground and jump or step back into *Chaturanga Dandasana* (22). Inhale into *Urdhva Mukha Svanasana* (23), exhale *Adho Mukha Svanasana* (15). Inhale, lunge forward (alternate legs each time) and look forward lifting the sternum (24), on exhale head to floor (25), on inhale look forward again (24), on exhale leg back. Repeat the lunge movements with the opposite leg straightaway on next inhale. Then having exhaled back into *Adho Mukha Svanasana*, inhale swing via plank into *Urdhva Mukha Svanasana* with the toes tucked under **(26)**, and from there spread the knees and bring the bum to your heels **(2)**. Place the forearms on the floor, elbows and hands in line and shoulder-width apart. Tuck toes under and lift into Elbow Dog **(27)**. Hold for at least three breaths. If you can, inhale both elbows off the floor evenly at the same time. Otherwise, exhale the knees to the floor and then inhale back into *Adho Mukha Svanasana*. Jump forward and inhale into *Ardha Uttanasana* **(21)**. Exhale *Uttanasana* **(20)**, inhale *Urdhva Hastasana* **(19)**, exhale *Samasthiti* **(8)**. Repeat, but this time do the Dolphin **(28)**, once you get into Elbow Dog **(27)**. Exhale, plunging the nose down to the gap between the thumbs and inhaling back up again.

Do at least four complete Lotus Mandala *Suryanamaskaras*.

STANDING POSES

(29) Step into Horse-Riding Stance. Feet are turned out at 45 degrees and a leg-length between the heels. Sink low, but the sitting bones must not go lower than the knees. Do the following shoulder-strengthening exercises in Horse-Riding Stance:

• **(30)** Bull's Horns. Bend the elbows, which must remain higher than shoulders, form fists, and begin making circles backwards and forwards with them. Imagine you are moving through a resistance, slowing the rotations down.

• Release the fists and like bench presses, exhale push down, and inhale pull up again, always working against resistence. Still ensure that the elbows remain higher than the shoulders.

• Straighten the arms and grab an invisible iron bar straight ahead of you. Now twist that bar, bending only the wrists, not the elbows. Grab it again on the in-breath with the opposite hand on top and again exhale twist. Repeat several times.

• Take the hands back in *namaste*. From there sweep down and take the arms to horizontal, as you straighten the legs, turning the toes in and the heels out.

Rotate the shoulders forward and place the hands into *namaste* behind the back. Inhale look up, opening the heart-space, exhale into

(31) *Prasarita Padottanasana*. Hold.

Inhale up and square the hips to the back of the room. You may need to shorten and widen your stance somewhat, and pull the back heel back. Inhale, look up, and exhale bend into

(32) *Parsvottanasana*.

Hold! Legs are straight, sacrum flat. Press the palms together.

Inhale, bring the torso vertical and look forward, fixing your *drishti*. Exhale, bend the front leg knee, inhale lift the back leg off, while straightening the standing leg for

(33) *Virabhadrasana 3*.

Flex the extended leg foot to help level the sacrum and stretch strongly into the heel.

Exhale the back foot down again and inhale up from there.

Swivel on the feet and swing the hips around, square now to the front. Repeat *Parsvottanasana* and Warrior 3 on this side. Turn the hips flat to the side, slide the fingers down the spine, extend into fingertips, and step into *Samastithi*.

Interlock the fingers and do wrist rotations in both directions.

ARM BALANCES

(Moon-day girls can practice coming up, but do not hold any inversion during this time of your monthly cycle.)

(35) *Pincha Mayurasana*

To come into the forearm balance, or *Pincha Mayurasana* ("Peacock's Tail-Feather Pose"), place the forearms shoulder-width apart on the mat. The tendency is for the elbows to slide apart and the hands to slide together. The balance also can be tricky. Therefore most people practice against the wall and use a brick and belt if necessary. (See Chapter 3, *Arm Balances*.) The *drishti* is between the thumbs.

(34) To come up into *Pincha Mayurasana*, stretch one leg up high on the in-breath. Start the out-breath and draw the second leg to the first, gently kicking it up if necessary. Once there (35), keep the legs together and stretch them to the sky. Press firmly into the arms. Grip *mula* and *uddhiyana bandha* strongly, in order to avoid collapsing into the lumbar. Sustain the strong, steady *ujaii* breath! Eventually you will work up to ten breaths.

(36) When you are confident in *Pincha Mayurasana*, variations such as the Half-Lotus Scorpion or even the Full Lotus Twist

(SEE LARGE ILL. ABOVE) become possible. The greater the arch in the back, the more you need to lift your head up to your toes. Come out the same way you went in, scissoring the legs. Beware not to hurt the toes. As the leg is circumscribing a considerable arch, it can come down with quite some vehemence.

(38) *Adho Mukha Vrikshasana*, or Dowward-Facing Tree (Handstand)

(37) Place the hands shoulder-width apart on the floor. If you are using a wall, place them about a hand-length from the wall. Your *drishti* is slightly ahead of the hands. Have the legs together and touching, as you inhale bend the knees, start the exhalation and bunny-hop up, so that you are bringing the pelvis over the shoulder-girdle. Push strongly through the arms, as you slowly straighten the legs and stretch them to the sky. Grip *mula* and *uddhiyana bandha* firmly, in order to avoid collapsing into the lumbar. Sustain the strong, steady *ujaii* breath! Eventually you will work up to ten breaths. Come out the same way you went in, slowly bending the knees to the chest and with conrol bringing the feet back to the floor.

FLOOR WORK

(29) Step back out into Horse-Riding Stance.

(39) Moving *Lutasana*, Spider Pose

Bend the knees and press the elbows against the inner knee. On the out-breath, straighten one leg, as you bend the opposite knee. Keep the feet flat on the ground, the chest open, never hunching. The *drishti* is on the straight-leg foot. Inhale back the center and exhale to the other side. At first straighten the legs between sides, but eventually keep the bum as low as possible throughout. Inhale on transit and exhale to the side.

Come back to center, place the hands or forearms on the floor and slowly slide the feet apart into

(40) *Samakonasana*, the side-splits

Keep the soles grounded, the pelvis in line with the feet and the thoracic region broad. Reinforce *mula bandha* to protect the groin. Hold for several long, steady *ujaii* breaths, relax and let gravity work for you.

If you are sufficiently far down in the splits, you may be able to slowly lower the sitting bones to the floor, but otherwise it is safer to just bend the knees and take yourself to sitting with the legs at a 90-degree angle for

(41) *Upavishta Konasana*

Exhale, bend forward, catching the outer edges of the feet if possible. The legs are gripped, knees and toes pointing up throughout. If it is hard for you to hinge from the hips in this forward bend, it may be beneficial to sit up on a block and pull the flesh of the sitting bones apart before you go forward. Hold.

Inhale out of *Upavishta Konasana* and take the back leg into a straddle for

(42) *Parighasana.*

Check that there is still a right angle at the groin, as you

reach in with the straight-leg arm and up with the bent-leg arm, looking past its fingertips. With the upwardly extended arm reach and perhaps catch the outer edge of the straight leg. The other hand grabs the inner edge. Enjoy this beautiful side-bend!

Inhale up and take the straddle leg to meet the straight leg. From there do *Parighasana* on the other side.

Inhale up and bring the legs together for

(43) *Dandasana*, the Staff Pose.

The spine is straight like a staff, the hands are beside the hips and the legs are gripped, pushing the backs of the knees and the heels into the ground.

(44) Inhale the arms up, interlocking the fingers. Hinging from the hips, lower the flat torso down in ten-degree increments on each out-breath. Sustain the work in the legs and keep the arms beside the ears, reaching far. Eventually this will take you into

(45) *Paschimottanasana.*

(46) From here do a half-*vinyasa*, crossing the legs and lifting yourself into *Lolasana* on the in-breath. Exhale head forward, legs shoot back into *Chatwari* **(22)**, inhale *Urdhva Mukha Svanasana* **(23)**, exhale *Adho Mukha Svanasana* **(15)**. Jump through and gently lower yourself back into *Dandasana* **(43)**.

Half Lotus Sequence:

Bend your left knee in tight and drop it out to the side. Scoop the foot by the ankle and gently lift the leg into Half-Lotus.

Support the knee with a block if necessary. Swing the left arm around the back and wrap index and middle finger around the big toe, coming into the forward bend with the free right arm. Some yogis may prefer to precede this by a gentle twist to the left to help reach the toe, but then you need to derotate. Otherwise, you could use a belt as a loop if you can't catch. Or just exhale forward with both arms into

(47) *Ardha Baddha Padma Paschimottanasana*

Hold and breathe, releasing but never forcing.

Inhale up from there. Exhale lower and release the arms. Inhale the left arm up and exhale, catch the outer edge of your right foot. Swing the right arm around the back and try to catch the left thigh or even the shin, looking past your right shoulder and twisting into

(48) *Matsyendrasana*

Open the sternum and pull the shoulder blades down the back. Deep, steady *ujaii* breathing. Enjoy the Lord of Fish Twist!

Release, and still preserving the left Half-Lotus leg if the hip is sufficiently open and the knee safe, bend the right leg and place the foot firmly on the ground. Reach forward and wrap the right arm around the right bent leg and catch the left hand behind your back. Exhale the head down towards the ground for

(49) *Marichiasana B*

For those whose hips are too tight or knees too fragile, *Marichiasana A* is more appropriate, where the left leg is kept straight.

(50) *Vatayanasana*, the Horse-Face Pose is only for those with a confident Lotus. Place the left knee on the floor, the right foot flat, beside and slightly in front of the foot. Cross the right arm over the left and then cross again, placing the hands in *namaste* prayer (Eagle arms). Push through the flat foot, draw up using *mula bandha*, stretch the figertips to the sky, and if you can, lift the *drishti* as well! Even when you are looking up, there is a pulling in and back of the chin with *jalandhara bandha*, which will give you further stability. Release.

Do a half-*vinyasa*, even preserving the Half Lotus leg up until *Adho Mukha Svanasana*, if you can.

Repeat the same sequence with the right leg in Half Lotus!

ABDOMINALS AND CORE

Lie on your back and raise the legs into

(51) *Urdhva Parsarita Padasana.*

Place the arms beside your head with the palms facing up. Drop the belly into the back and flatten the back to the ground. Extend into the balls of the feet, as you exhale the legs to 80 degrees. Inhale deeply and on the out-breath again lower to 70 degrees. Again breathe in.

(52) Abdominal supine leg work

Keep slowly lowering the legs in 10 degree increments on the exhalations, until they are all the way down. Ensure that the whole back remains grounded, by strongly gripping the *bandhas* and engaging the legs!

Sit up. Place the feet hip-width and parallel and the hands shoulder-width behind you with the fingers pointing forward and lift up into

(53) Table-Top Pose
Ensure that the heels are beneath the knees and the hands beneath the shoulders. Flatten out the top. Snuggle one sole firmly into the ground and then raise the other leg up for the

(54) One-Legged Table-Top Pose
Make sure you do not collapse the hip. Hold for at least five breaths on each side, never allowing the supporting leg foot to slide.

BACKBENDS

Do a half-*vinyasa* and from *Adho Mukha Svanasana*, inhale into Plank Pose **(55)**, exhale into *Chatwari* **(22)** and lie down on your belly.
Bend your knees and catch the ankles. Make sure you are turning the shoulders out, not in! Have the big toes touching and the knees squeezing in towards each other to safeguard the lumbar, as you lift up into

(56) *Dhanurasana*, the Bow
Stretch the tips of toes to the sky, lift the chest and the gaze, but keep the back of the neck long. Hold and preserve the deep steady *ujaii* pranayama right through the backbending section.
Once you've released, turn your face to the side, shake your hips out to jiggle the spine.

Then move the legs together again, bend the knees, catch the inner ankles, flex the feet and again lift up into this

(59) *Dhanurasana* variation and breathe.
Release. Turn the face the other way and again relieve the back by shaking the hips out.
Either just roll over onto your back or do a half-*vinyasa* and lie down.
Bend the knees and place the feet hip-width apart and parallel. Place the hands beneath the shoulders and keeping the elbows above the wrists, on the exhalation lift up into

(58) *Urdhva Dhanurasana.*
Make sure that the feet don't splay, so keep the heels in. Inhale, look to the sky, and lift the heart space, carefully increasing the pressure from the legs, exhale hang the head, but keep that opening.
Do at least five breaths here and then lower the crown of the head back to the ground.
From here once again lift into the Upward Bow Pose **(58)**. Explore entering the asana on the inhalation if there is sufficient strength. Imagine the sky was a magnet drawing you up, and you simply need to expand into its forcefield. Transit in and out smoothly, carefully monitoring the quality of your breath. Work up to four times, five breaths. The lie down for the

(59) Supine Eagle Twist.
Lay the arms by the side perpendicular to your body, palms up. Raise the legs and cross the right leg over the left, cross

the legs again, hooking the foot. Lower the legs over to the right, whilst turning your gaze to the left and drawing the left shoulder blade to the ground. Hold and breathe into the twist, releasing into gravity.

Inhale the legs up. Uncross on the out-breath and then on the in-breath, set up the eagle legs the opposite way and exhale them to the left, while turning the head to the right and drawing the right shoulder blade into the ground. Hold. Inhale up, untwist the legs. From here you can do *Chakrasana*, the backward roll, into *Balasana* (1) and (2) at the back of the mat, but please be extremely careful with your neck, holding an exaggerated *jalandhara bandha*, chin glued to the sternum. Also, work with the breath and with momentum and make yourself compact like a ball, knees bent into the body and legs together.

FINISHING & INVERSIONS

From here you are in the perfect position to set up for (60) *Shirsasana*, the Headstand

Moon-day girls, skip all long-held inversions or go into the menstrual poses instead. (See Chapter 5.)

Kneeling, place the elbows shoulder-width apart on the ground and don't let them slide apart. Interlock the hands, but keep the thumbs apart and lay the forearms firmly on the ground. If you are using a wall, the interlaced fingers should be right up against it. Place the crown of the head on the floor and the back of the head into the cradle of your hands. Then bring the thumb-tips to touch. Tuck your toes under and walk the pelvis above the shoulder-girdle. Eventually the legs will rise up straight and together, but beginners may need to hop up and then slowly straighten the legs. A good headstand preserves all the qualities of the Mountain Pose (8). *Bandhas* engaged, never collapsing into the lower back. Legs are firm reaching to the sky. Shoulders are away from the ears, leaving the neck free. *Ujaii* breath calm and strong.

Parivrittaikapada Shirsasana (61)

Whilst extending strongly into the balls of the feet, slowly move the left leg forward and the right leg back, scissoring the legs. Keep the cohesion at the pelvis and do not collapse the spine. On the exhalation, gently rotate to the right, never losing the *ujaii* breath. Hold and then slowly come back to center and bring the legs together. Then scissor the left leg forward and the right leg back and exhale twist to the left. Hold and come back to centre and bring the legs together. Settle back into the central alignment of *Shirsasana* (60) and then slowly spread your legs on the in-breath, and exhale bend the knees bringing the soles of the feet together for *Konasana* in *Shirsasana*. (62) Hold.

Finally bring the knees together slowly and gently lower the legs to the ground back into *Balasana* (1) and (2). Do not pull your head up, but rest here for a good few breaths, until the neck feels like an integral part of the spine again. Then inhale and sit up.

Place the hands on the ground beside the knees. Inhale, lift the body off the ground, gripping the *bandhas* strongly and exhale cross the legs and bring them through, so you end up sitting down.

From here if you can do so safely, take yourself into
(63) *Padmasana*, the Lotus.
Otherwise, come into *Sukhasana*, simple crossed legs. Place the hands behind you and keeping the knees grounded, look up and open the heart space for
(64) Yoga Mudra.
From here come back up, placing the hands in *jnana* mudra on the knees, index and middle finger touching **(63)**. Find that strong, steady *ujaii* breath again, the inner alignment of the *bandhas* to prepare yourself for
(65) *Utpluthih*.
With the hands flat beside your hips, lift your entire body off the ground. This is far more difficult in the simple cross-legged position than in the Lotus, so do not feel concerned if you can't hold it for as long as those yogis in *Padmasana*. Keeping the body off the floor, begin the fire breath, pushing the abdomen back for a strong exhalation, drawing it out again for a sharp inhalation. Start with a low breath count, but eventually work up to one hundred.

RELAXATION

Lower down and go straight in to the relaxation in
(66) *Savasana*, the Corpse Pose

Consciously "unlock" the *bandhas*, softening the inner body. Return from *ujaii* to soundless, relaxed abdominal breathing. Float in the pranic intoxication, allowing every single cell of the body to be cushioned in its benevolent, healing embrace. Hold for as long as you like, but at least five minutes is advisable. Then wiggle your fingers and toes to bring yourself back to your physical self, bend the knees and roll onto your right-hand side. From there without disturbing the peace, gently take yourself up to sitting.
Namaste!

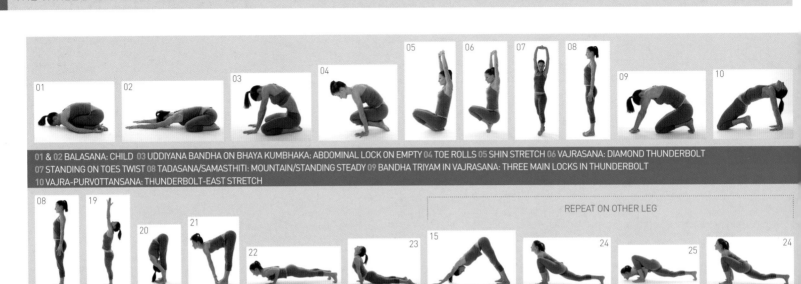

01 & 02 BALASANA: CHILD 03 UDDIYANA BANDHA ON BHAYA KUMBHAKA: ABDOMINAL LOCK ON EMPTY 04 TOE ROLLS 05 SHIN STRETCH 06 VAJRASANA: DIAMOND THUNDERBOLT
07 STANDING ON TOES TWIST 08 TADASANA/SAMASTHITI: MOUNTAIN/STANDING STEADY 09 BANDHA TRIYAM IN VAJRASANA: THREE MAIN LOCKS IN THUNDERBOLT
10 VAJRA-PURVOTTANSANA: THUNDERBOLT-EAST STRETCH

REPEAT ON OTHER LEG

19 URDHVA HASTASANA: UPWARD EXTENDED ARMS 20 UTTANASANA: STANDING FORWARD BEND 21 ARDHA UTTANASANA: HALF STANDING FORWARD BEND
22 CHATURANGA DANDASANA: FOUR-LIMBED ROD (PRESS-UP POSE) 23 URDVHA MUKHA SVANASANA: UPWARD-FACING DOG 24 LUNGE UP 25 LUNGE DOWN

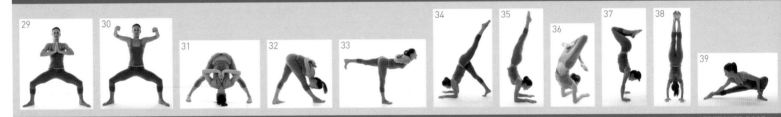

29 ASHVAROHINASANA: HORSE-RIDING STANCE 30 HORSE WITH BULL'S HORNS 31 PRASARITA PADOTTANASANA: INTENSE SPREAD LEG STRETCH 32 PARSVOTTANASANA: LATERAL STRETCHED POSE
33 VIRABHADRASANA 3: WARRIOR 3 34 PINCHAMAYURASANA PREP 35 PINCHAMAYURASANA: PEACOCK'S FEATHER 36 ARDHA PADMA VRISCHIKASANA: HALF LOTUS SCORPION
37 HANDSTAND BUNNY HOP 38 ADHO MUKHA VRIKSHASANA: DOWNWARD-FACING TREE (HANDSTAND) 39 LUTASANA: SPIDER

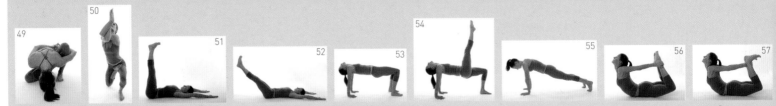

49 MARICHIASANA B: SAGE MARICHI 50 VATAYANASANA: HORSE-FACE 51 URDVHA PRASARITA PADASANA: UPWARD EXTENDED LEG POSE 52 ABDOMINAL SUPINE LEG WORK
53 BHARMANASANA: TABLE-TOP 54 EKA PADA BHARMANASANA: ONE-LEGGED TABLE-TOP 55 PLANK 56 DHANURASANA: BOW 57 DHANURASANA VARIATION

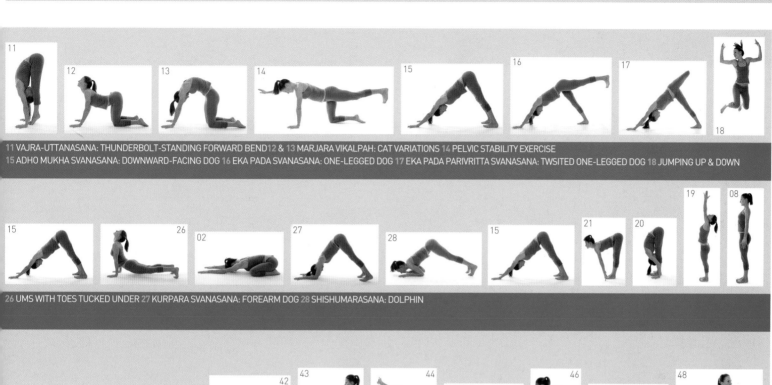

11 VAJRA-UTTANASANA: THUNDERBOLT-STANDING FORWARD BEND 12 & 13 MARJARA VIKALPAH: CAT VARIATIONS 14 PELVIC STABILITY EXERCISE
15 ADHO MUKHA SVANASANA: DOWNWARD-FACING DOG 16 EKA PADA SVANASANA: ONE-LEGGED DOG 17 EKA PADA PARIVRITTA SVANASANA: TWSITED ONE-LEGGED DOG 18 JUMPING UP & DOWN

26 UMS WITH TOES TUCKED UNDER 27 KURPARA SVANASANA: FOREARM DOG 28 SHISHUMARASANA: DOLPHIN

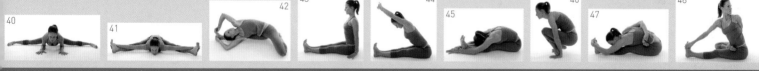

40 SAMAKONASANA: GREAT ANGLE (SIDE SPLITS) 41 UPAVISHTA KONASANA: SEATED ANGLE POSE 42 PARIGHASANA: GATE 43 DANDASANA: ROD
44 ARDHA PASCHIMOTTANASANA: HALF WEST STRETCH 45 PASCHIMOTTANASANA: WEST STRETCH (SEATED FORWARD BEND) 46 LOLASANA: EARRING
47 ARDHA BADHA PADMA PASCHIMOTTANASANA: HALF BOUND LOTUS FORWARD BEND 48 MATSUYENDRASANA: LORD OF FISH

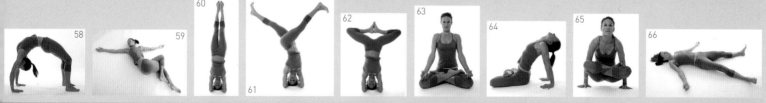

58 URDVHA DHANURASANA: UPWARD BOW 59 SUPTA PARIVRITTA GARUDASANA: SUPINE EAGLE TWIST 60 SHIRSASANA: HEADSTAND 61 KONASANA IN SHIRSASANA: ANGLE IN HEADSTAND
62 PARIVRITTAIKAPADA SHIRSASANA: ROTATED SPLIT LEG HEADSTAND 63 PADMASANA: LOTUS 64 YOGA MUDRA: SEAL OF UNION 65 UTPLUTHIH: UPROOTING 66 SHAVASANA: CORPSE

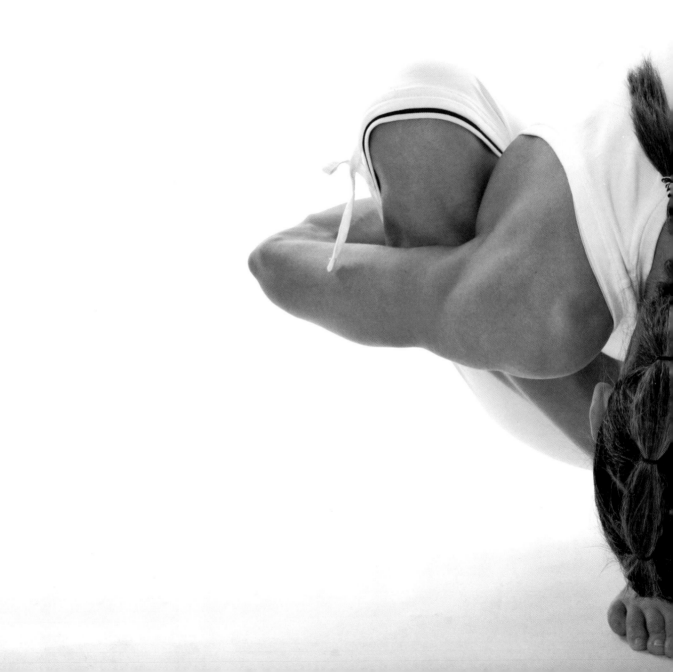

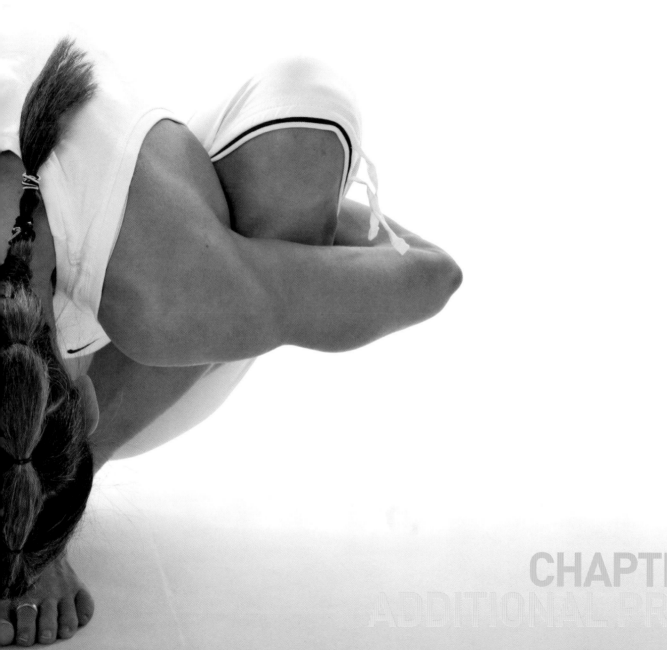

PURE PRANAYAMA

We all move our bodies consciously at some point or other, but how often do we consciously exercise our way of breathing? Although breathing exercises look easier to perform than the average yoga posture, beware! In *pranayama*, we are dealing with the very essence of life and such a practice should be approached with great care. Our breath has a considerable impact on our health, psychological disposition, and state of mind.

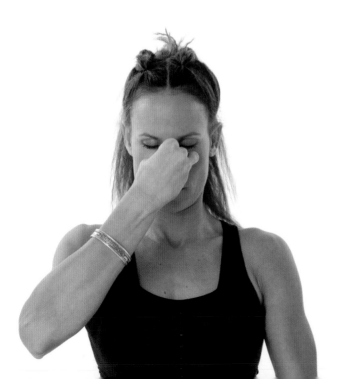

The word *pranayama* means both control (*yama*) and extension (*ayama*) of prana (vital life force). Hence the word indicates the ability to withhold the breath, as well as the capacity to expand one's intake of breath through the lungs, hereby maximizing the assimilation of prana.

The three essential building blocks of pranyama are: inhalation (*puraka*), exhalation (*rechaka*), and retention (*kumbhaka*). The latter can be further divided into *antara kumbhaka* (inhalation retention) and *bhaya* (or *bahir*) *kumbhaka* (exhalation retention). Out of these an endless array of exercises can be constructed that have distinctly varying effects. In this chapter I will introduce you to some of the basic *pranayamas*. I would recommend you watch the Pranayama section of the accompanying Quantum Yoga DVD for further clarification. All of these exercises I learned from my teacher Clive Sheridan and I would advise you to seek the direct guidance of a qualified teacher in learning this science. If you do not have this luxury, there are a few things you need to pay attention to. If you suffer from hypertension, are pregnant or have bouts of vertigo, it is advisable to avoid the retentions altogether. Just stick to very simple pranayama such as *nadi shodana*. Although you are of course working towards increasing your ability to control the breath, never let excess pressure build up. Just like with asana, so with *pranayama* your approach should be one of balancing effort (*sthira*) with ease (*sukha*). Be patient and progress slowly but consistently. Also accept that there will be days when it seems you have gone a few steps back. The breath never lies. If you are intoxicated, emotionally drained, or hyped up, or your mind is excessively busy, this will translate into a lower quality of your breath. Naturally, the more regular and solid your asana and pranayama practice, the less likely it is that outer circumstances will take you into that state in the first place.

Our tendency to shallow breath, especially when we find ourselves in stressful situations, means that we are not exploiting our true energetic capacity, especially when we most need it! The volume of our tidal breath lags well behind our vital capacity. When breathing normally, the tidal air is only very slowly exchanged, so there is always a certain measure of "stale" air in our lungs. Through regular practice of *pranayama*, the body has access to more oxygen-rich fresh air. It is no wonder therefore, that it leads to higher levels of vitality and joy. If you love asana practice, watch how it improves once you also begin doing specific *pranayama* exercises regularly.

POSTURE IN PRANAYAMA

As in meditation (see Chapter 3, *Meditation*), so in pranayama, a good upright posture, which promotes a relaxed attitude whilst remaining fully alert, will support focus and the

capacity to assimilate and harness prana. *Mula* and *jalandhara bandha* (root and chin lock) should ideally be engaged throughout your *pranayama* practice. A full *uddhiyana bandha* is only applied in certain cases, although you are often manipulating the flow of prana using the abdominal muscles, for instance by pumping the navel as described in the first *pranayama* below. However, your posture should ensure that the abdomen never collapses forward, which would constrict the lumbar region and overarch the back. Remember that the spine must remain upright, that the seat needs to be firm, the shoulders relaxed, the chest open, and the chin in.

BASIC PRANAYAMAS

UJAII PRANAYAMA (VICTORIOUS BREATH)—FOCUSING AND EMPOWERING

Ujaii is explained in the *Sublimatio* section, as a lengthening, deepening and sharpening of the nasal breath through a contraction at the back of the throat, resulting in a gentle rasping sound. All three *bandhas* are gently engaged. Simply sitting and breathing in *ujaii* is particularly good on days when there is great mental and emotional unrest, to the point where concentration seems impossible. Its soothing sound will help you pull everything together and find your center again. As you sit and breathe in this manner, feel how on the inhalation, through the engagement of *uddiyana bandha*, the ribcage expands in all directions, front, sides and back.

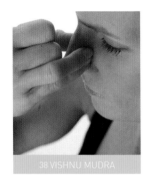

38 VISHNU MUDRA

This widening of your torso gives you a powerful sense of Shakti's generative power, Mother Earth energy coming in and providing. On the exhalation, as the diaphragm lifts and everything hugs in and lengthens, gently reinforce the *bandhas* pulling up from your root. Allow anything you no longer need and have been unnecessarily holding, to sink into the ground and dissolve into the breath. Visualize that central rod of light, the *sushumna nadi*, and lay the energy that you have pulled up from muladhara chakra at the feet of Shiva in the seat of wisdom at the third eye. From *ajna* chakra thus join the silent observer and become witness to the play of life, as communicated by the breath.

AGNI SARI (FIRE BREATH)
CLEANSING

Agni Sari primarily clears phlegm from the nasal passage (therefore have some tissue paper handy!). To do this *pranayama* you need to position one hand in Vishnu mudra, which is like forming a nose-clamp with your hand
(SEE ILL.38). The other hand can remain in *jnana* mudra, with tip of thumb and index finger touching. Mudras are "seals" that fix the particular attitude you are assuming and create energy circuits in the body. (See *Mudra* section below for symbolism.)

To do Vishnu mudra, curl index and middle finger in, as you will not be using those, and place the tip of your thumb on one side of the nose, and the tip of the ring and pinkie finger on the other side. Position them just where the bony bit of the nose ends and the fleshy bit starts. There you will only have to apply very gentle pressure to manipulate the nasal passage. In fact, you don't ever really need to lift these fingers completely off the nose. Instead rotate the wrist slightly to move from one side to the other. Beware not to apply too much pressure, as this will cause you to pull the head over to the side, which would create a kink in your energy flow, as the neck is very much part of the spine. And it is along the spine that the sushumna nadi, the central channel, flows.

For *agni sari*, we do twenty breaths on the left, twenty on the right, and then twenty with both nostrils. The breaths are vigorous and sharp, generated by the regular pumping of the navel. As you breathe out, the navel pulls back, as you breathe in, it draws out. Unlike in *kapalabhati pranayama*, described below, where you are primarily focusing on the exhalation, here both parts, *rechaka* and *puraka*, should be strong.

Start with a slow exhalation on the left nostril, and then do twenty short sharp breaths pumping from the navel. Change sides after the last inhalation. Release a long exhalation from the right nostril and again do twenty short sharp breaths pumping from the navel, ending with the in-breath. Place the hand down in *jynan* mudra, exhale from both nostrils and again do twenty breaths, in-out.

From here do one *ujaii* breath, and return to relaxed abdominal breathing.

Normally I do three rounds of *agni sari* in one session.

KAPALABHATI ("SHINING SKULL")
INVIGORATING AND CLEANSING

This *pranayama* complements the next one (*bandha triyam* on *bhaya kumbhaka*) and the two are often done together. It is not appropriate for moon-day girls or pregnant women. Also, if you have recently had a hernia or any other lesion of the abdominal wall, you should wait until the wound is completely healed up before you attempt this.

Place your palms on your knees to give you greater stability as you can push against the legs when engaging the three locks. Begin by inhaling deeply and then rapidly and vigorously pumping the belly, exhaling with each pump, until your lungs are empty. The feeling is one of bouncing the diaphragm.

BANDHA TRIYAM ON BHAYA KUMBHAKA
STRENGTHENING AND ALIGNING

Now inhale completely again and then sticking your tongue out exhale fully in Lion Breath. There are versions of the Lion's Breath that are done very vigorously and sharply, with the tongue pointed, the eyes wide open and focused on the third eye (*shambhavi* mudra), which are particularly useful when cleansing the throat and release of pent up emotion is necessary. Here, however, we are talking about a much deeper and lower lion's breath, more like a quiet roar than a hiss. Once you are completely empty, hold the breath out and release back into the vacuum you have created through *bhaya kumbhaka*, the exhalation retention. *Bandha triyam* engages the inner musculature by drawing in and up, initiating what could be described as an implosion into and through oneself. It feels as though you had let all the air out of a container, which you are now vacuum-packing.

Bhandha triyam echoes the mental experience you have in meditation, the true focus of your entire attention on one point. Eventually it feels a bit like you are sucking the entirety of your being through an impossibly tight loophole. This loophole is the gateway to infinity, a level of consciousness the thought-mind cannot access. And so *bandha triyam*, with the integrity and coalescence it establishes, represents your access route to a way of posture, and in conjunction with ujaii breathing a way of movement, that ensures a perfect flow of prana along sushumna nadi. The three bandhas are *mula bandha*, the root lock; uddhiyana bandha, the abdominal lock; and jalandhara bandha, the chin lock. Naturally in this exercise we are gripping them in an exaggerated fashion, so as to bring the awareness into these parts, tone the muscles, and massage the organs. Remember that the body is made out of spongy tissue and that like a sponge, when you release the contraction, the blood then flows more readily into all parts and brings with it oxygen and *prana*. Once you have released the intense grip of the *bandhas*, you will be left with just a gentle engagement that ensures a steady and pleasant seat, *Sthira sukham asanam*. Remember that the *bandhas* must be released, *before* inhaling, so that the breath flows in smooth.

Generally, and this goes for all *kumbhaka* retentions, in or out, you can judge how long you should be holding by the quality of the out- or in-breath that follows, which should be smooth and controlled. If this is not the case, you have held the retention for too long. Reduce the time and increase it slowly from there.

BHASTRIKA (BELLOWS BREATH)
INCREASES LUNG CAPACITY AND STIMULATES

Bhastrika results in a distinctly cosmic state, though when overdone, it can increase the blood pressure to such an extent that the practitioner may feel quite dizzy. In this case you should reduce the length of the retention and the number of repetitions should be left to a minimum until one is more established in this exercise. Also, check that *jalandhara bandha* and *mula bandha* are engaged properly, as especially the former keeps the blood pressure down. Finally, a technique I've developed is to swallow if ever I feel spaced out, and strangely it seems to take me back down to earth.

Sitting in a comfortable but stable position, the hands in *jnana* mudra on the knees, begin by drawing fifteen strong and sharp breaths right up into the chest and heart space. As you pull up, reinforce *mula bandha*. After the fifteenth breath, exhale completely and then inhale as deeply as you can into the chest and the heart region and hold the breath in. Again grip *mula* and *jalandhara bandha* firmly. Initiate the slow, steady exhalation well before you feel any pressure in the head. Make sure to empty yourself out completely, before returning to relaxed abdominal breathing. Remember again that the correct length for you to be holding the retention can be monitored by the quality of the exhalation that follows. In other words, if you are *not* able to exhale in a controlled and smooth fashion, this is a clear indication that you have held the retention for too long. Naturally, you are progressively increasing your lung capacity and your ability to hold the breath in, but this must be undertaken very slowly and with great patience. Anybody who ignores this basic instruction is quite simply gambling with life itself. Prana is the essence of life and should be approached with great respect. Breath control cannot be learned overnight, so please view this as a long, slow, and steady journey, which will progressively lead to greater health and vitality, the capacity to still your thoughts and eventually bring lasting inner peace. Breath control is mind control, as the message of the ancient sages of yoga goes, but not the other way around. If the ego-mind projects and imposes on the system practices the body is not yet ready for, this can severely backfire, both in the domain of asana, but even more so with *pranayama*.

Once you have returned to relaxed abdominal breathing, enjoy the inner radiance and the pranic intoxication *antara kumbhaka* brings. Visualise the prana like the rays of the sun emanating from the solar plexus, out through the *nadis*, shining forth like a bright halo of light enveloping your entire being. Sit like this in stillness, until you feel very calm again and then initiate another round. Do three rounds to start with, but never more than five in a single sitting.

NADI SHODANA (CLEANSING OF THE NADIS)
BALANCING

Nadi shodana is the most important of the *pranayamas*. Should you have time for only one, *nadi shodana* is the exercise you should do. It is a continuous *pranayama* and Vishnu mudra is held throughout. Therefore, be extra cautious that you do not press the fingers too firmly against the nose, thereby pulling the head to the side. To check whether this is the case, you can bend the neck a bit more and place the chin into the jugular notch, to assure that it is in a central positioning. Also, make sure that you are not pressing the elbow of the Vishnu mudra arm against the chest, thereby constricting the openness of the lungs. As this can be a challenging position to hold the arm in for an extended amount of time, there is a

tendency to stiffen the shoulder. Should this be the case, try changing sides and using the other arm.

Having assumed a comfortable and upright position, place the hand in Vishnu mudra on the nose and begin with a slow steady exhalation on the left nostril, counting to ten in your head. Inhale through the left nostril again to the count of ten. Change sides and exhale on the right nostril, counting to ten. Then inhale through right on ten. Change sides and begin the next round with *rechaka* through the left nostril, always keeping up the same count. If ten is too difficult and you find that you are straining, take the count down to eight or even five. If it is too easy, take it up to twelve, then fifteen and eventually twenty. However take your time, as the success of your *nadi shodana* can be judged by the continuous smooth quality of the breath. Remember that you are always changing sides when the lungs are full, after the inhalation.

The essence of *nadi shodana* is balance. Bear this is mind, always ensuring that all elements are even, same length left to right nostril, same length *puraka* and *rechaka*. Furthermore, the intensity of the breath should be even throughout, neither greedy at the beginning nor forced at the end of the in- or out-breath.

Continue with the *nadi shodana* count, but then consciously allow the numbers to drop away and go on your feeling alone, breathing for even lengths. Always end the exercise with the exhalation on the left nostril. The symmetric *pranayamas* begin and end with the rechaka on the left nostril. Then take the hand back down into *jnana* mudra, do one more full *ujaii* breath and from there return to relaxed abdominal breathing.

These are the pranayamas I practice almost daily. Time permitting, I usually add on a choice of one of the below at the end. In total, I therefore usually sit for pranayama for about forty-five minutes to an hour.

OTHER PRANAYAMAS:

ANULOMA

Anuloma is slightly more complicated than the pranayamas described above, as it is asymmetric in its breath count. It is usually done on a seven-five-ten rhythm. As always when you begin a *pranayama* exercise, check that your posture is good. Once satisfied, start counting to seven as you inhale through both nostrils. Hold the breath in on the count of five. Take the hand up into Vishnu mudra and slowly exhale through the left nostril for ten. Bring the hand back down again, inhale on seven through both nostrils, and hold *antara kumbhaka* for five. Bring the hand up into Vishnu mudra and exhale through

the right nostril for ten. Continue with the anuloma, always ensuring that *mula* and *jalandhara bandha*, root and chin lock, are gently engaged. Once you are more confident in the exercise you can take the count up to ten-seven-fourteen, but again slow progress is better than rushed, forced haste.

As in the *nadi shodana*, eventually allow the numbers to drop away and go on your feeling alone: medium-length *puraka*, short *antara kumbhaka*, and long *rechaka* on alternate nostrils. Always end the exercise with the exhalation on the right nostril. The asymmetric *pranayamas* begin with rechaka on the left nostril and end with rechaka on the right nostril. Then take the hand back down into *jnana* mudra, do one more full *ujaii* breath and from there return to relaxed abdominal breathing.

PRATILOMA

Pratiloma literally means "going against the grain," which describes the conscious effort not to release all air out of the body at once, as would be our natural tendency on the exhalation. In *pratiloma*, the breath is inhaled and then exhaled in three equal parts, holding for an even amount of counts between each section. You empty yourself from top to bottom, paying good attention to the sensation of release in the respective parts of the body. Then you inhale fully, exhale completely, inhale fully again, and start the next round. Begin by doing three rounds in one session and work your way slowly up to five.

VILOMA

Viloma can be done sitting upright, but I find that this *pranayama's* expansive effect is most effective when lying down in *Supta Baddha Konasana*, the Supine Bound Angle Pose. *Supta Baddha Konasana* allows the whole body to unfold, especially when done over a bolster or rolled-up blanket, making it the perfect receptacle for prana. *Viloma* is not appropriate if you suffer from high blood pressure. It is very good for regulating pitta and strengthening the inhalation. Hence, it is practiced at the beginning of the Heroes Sequence. *Supta Baddha Konasana* further supports the cooling aspect. I have also found it very effective against constipation.

In *viloma*, the breath is exhaled completely and the inhalation is split into three even parts. It helps to visualize the body as a vessel or pot, into which water is being poured in three even portions from bottom to top, until it is completely full to the rim. Thus begin by drawing the breath into the lower realm of the body, below the belly button, and hold for five counts. Then draw the second third of the inhalation into the middle torso below the solar plexus and hold for five. Feel the expansion of the rib cage at the sides and in the back as well.

Then draw the final third of the inhalation into the chest and heart region until you are completely full like a balloon that is about to burst. Hold the breath for five counts and then slowly and steadily exhale until you are completely empty. Inhale fully, exhale normally, inhale normally again, and then exhale, emptying yourself out completely. From that emptiness, begin the second round of the *viloma pranayama*. Start by doing three rounds and work up to five.

SAMAVRTTI

Samavrtti means "even parts." The breath is split into four even parts: *puraka* (inhalation), *antara kumbhaka* (inhalation retention), *rechaka* (exhalation), and *bhaya kumbhaka* (exhalation retention). The count is up to you, but again bear in mind never to be forceful, which would strain the nervous system and tax the body.

VISAMAVRTTI

Visamavrtti means "uneven parts." Like in *samavrtti*, the breath is split into its four parts (*puraka*, *antara kumbhaka*, *rechaka*, and *bhaya kumbhaka*), but they are deliberately uneven. This requires concentration and the capacity to adjust to the varying lengths.

SITALI

Sitali, or "cooling breath," is particularly useful when *pitta* is strong. It is done by forming a funnel with the tongue. (SEE ILL.39) Some people's genetic make-up does not allow for this ability, in which case one can just lay the tongue flat along the bottom lip. Inhaling through the funnel of the tongue cools the breath. The out-breath is slow and steady through the nose. Do this continuously and embrace the cooling sensation, allowing it in turn to chill your attitude and temper any passionate feelings that may have been getting in the way of your *chitta prasadanam*, or "innate serenity."

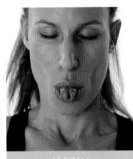

39 SITALI

BRAHMARI

Brahmari, or "the bumblebee," uses sound to yoke the senses and still the thoughts. One inhales through the nose, but exhales through the mouth with closed, soft lips, thereby making a gently buzzing sound. This *pranayama* is done continuously. The effect of *brahmari* can be strengthened by doing it in *yoni* mudra. (SEE ILL.40) The *yoni* symbolizes the feminine principle in nature, and in ancient cultures was symbolized by the shape of a round stone, into the center of which an indentation was carved. *Yoni* mudra represents the practice of *pratyahara*, or "sense withdrawal" (fifth Limb of Yoga). The tips of the pinkie fngers are placed at the edge of the mouth (nonspeaking), the ring fingers under the nose, without actually closing the nostril off (nonsmelling),

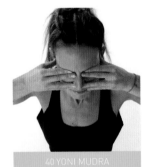

40 YONI MUDRA

the middle and index fingers are placed on the eyelids (nonseeing), and the thumbs close the ears (nonhearing). With *yoni* mudra the buzzing of the *brahmari pranayama* seems to envelop the entirety of your being and your thoughts easily dissolve into it (nonthinking).

Savasana, the Corpse Pose, should always be practiced after a long *pranayama* sitting. For most people, even if they do not realize it at the time, *pranayama* is far more challenging than asana. Also, as with asana, the full healing and rejuvenating effect of the *pranayama* is only really allowed to sink in and take effect if the mind, and with it action resulting from volition, is put to rest and the body is placed in a state of total relaxation. You won't necessarily be able to shut down all thought processes, but it is the act of consciously surrendering and allowing for things to happen to you that heightens our receptivity. It is therefore extremely important to do so after your efforts.

I am often asked, in what order should asana, *pranayama*, and meditation be practiced? As ever it all depends on the individual circumstances, one's personal aspirations and needs, but most importantly on the time of day. How I go about ordering "the limbs" is listed below.

Morning: Start with seated mediation while the mind is relatively still. Follow with a gentle Sublimatio. Then sit for *pranayama*. Perhaps then have a hot drink. Complete practice with asana.

Daytime: Start with *pranayama*, then asana, then meditation. Only rarely do people take time out in the day for yoga practice, as there is always a reason or distraction. Don't let your mind play tricks on you! It doesn't matter if you've recently eaten, you're not wearing the right clothes, or you may end up a bit sweaty and won't have time for a shower. I would say that if this is the only chunk of time you can make available for your yoga practice, don't make excuses, just do it. Decide how much time you've got, switch all telephones and other distracting devices off, and make a space for practice. If you think you have a million things left to do that you will forget, make a quick list and then put it away for later. Be ruthless and once you have started, don't let anything lure you away from your mat, even the fact that you may not have a mat and be doing it on the floor. The importance is to keep up your regular yoga practice. It should become like brushing your teeth or eating. Yoga is spiritual hygiene and should happen daily.

Evening: Start with asana, followed by *pranayama* and final meditation.

RESTORATIVE, MENSTRUAL AND PREGNANCY QUANTUM YOGA PRACTICE

The Ashtavakra Gita recounts an illustrative tale of a young boy named Ashtavakra, who was born deformed by eight (ashta) limbs (vakra) due to a curse his late father unthinkingly uttered in a fit of anger. Ashtavakra was raised into an intelligent child by his grandfather. Despite his limitations and the chiding comments he receives from all onlookers, the cripple bravely volunteeres to enter into debate with the great sage Bandhi. Losing the debate means Asthavakra will be drowned—a fate his father has already met with. Ashtavakra wins the debate and Bandhi finally discloses his true identity. He is the son of Varuna, the god of water, who sent him to bring sages to his court. The sages are then released from Varuna's underwater kingdom and Ashtavakra is reunited with his father. Furthermore, one dip in the water lifts the curse and Ashtavakra transforms into a handsome man.

Ashtavakra's story carries the message that through courage, persistence, and right knowledge, physical or mental handicaps are not in themselves limitations to success and fulfillment in life. Quantum Yoga is designed precisely to allow you to establish a yoga practice that is perfectly suited for you. This does not mean that you are working around your weaknesses, but with them. The objective is always to heal, strengthen, and transcend. If you only stay within the comfort zone of your strengths, they will become your weaknesses. Therefore lovingly and patiently focus on any deficiencies and reclaim your true form!

No matter how careful we are, weaknesses and restrictions will eventually creep up in our practice. This is no reason for worry. Yoga is designed to cleanse and transform, restoring the body to its true state of ease and power. The deeper we work into it, the more areas of resistance we are going to encounter. This will happen on the physical, the pranic, and the mental level in the course of our spiritual journey. I would say for asana what my teacher Clive Sheridan recommends in regards to disturbing thoughts in the context of meditation, "Welcome the uninvited guests!" Do not stop practicing altogether, but don't ignore pain either. I have already discussed in the Introduction through Chapter 3 how to differentiate between pain that could potentially lead to injury, as opposed to temporary discomfort that is an indication of expanding our range of physical experience.

ASHTAVAKRASANA

A detailed discussion of injuries and ailments goes beyond the scope of this book, but my aim is to give you some general advice in candidly conversing and constructively dealing with your body-mind, as well as that of others if you are teaching or simply guiding friends. I give myself or my students a restorative practice either if illness is coming and it is too late to simply sweat it out, or if it is still the early period of recovery. Once the state of sickness is actually there, the body will indicate it needs rest and this should be honored. Plenty of sleep is usually the answer and if you are established in a Quantum Yoga practice, the body's immune system should be strong enough to fend off almost any attack. Should you require medical assistance, if you have access to holistic practitioners, especially those working with Ayurvedic principles, this will be most in line with the yoga you are practicing.

Props take on additional significance in a restorative practice. What we are trying to do here is get the usual benefits of yoga asana, but without having to work the muscles in order to avoid any further depletion or strain. When fully supported, the body is invited to release totally into the poses. In this way they can also be held for a longer period of time. Check for the energetic effect in the respective groupings of the poses. With sufficient skill and imagination, you can support almost any pose using props. Below I will show you the two poses that I find most beneficial for body, heart, and mind in a restorative practice. Sometimes you cannot be sure of the psychosomatic causes of illness and many times the system is just calling out for nurture. I usually precede these restorative practices with a gentle Sublimatio, awakening the spine, rotating the joints, and opening the hips. Then I'll often do *viloma pranayama* in *Supta Baddha Konasana* (except in cases of hypertension) to increase prana and invite its healing power (see Pranyama section and the beginning of the Heroes sequence).

BACKBEND OVER THE CHAIR

Simple folding chairs are ideal for this restorative exercise. For bigger people, the backrest may need to be removed. Fold up a yoga mat in four and lay it over the chair seat. Place the chair about one and a half feet (half a meter) away from the wall, so that its back faces the wall. Climb into it, so that you are seated on it with your legs through the gap beneath the backrest. If it is awkward to climb into it this way, remember that for the most part these chairs are pretty light, so you can actually pick it up and put it on like you would a pair of trousers. Place the balls of your feet on the skirting board (or if there isn't one, just the bottom edge of the wall) hip-width apart, and wiggle your pelvis further through, as you lie back over the chair and thread your arms past the inside of the front chair legs, grabbing hold of the back chair legs with each hand (SEE ILL.41). As you do so, push the balls of the feet against the wall so your legs can straighten, as the chair slides along the floor into the correct position for you. Be mindful to keep the balls of feet in steady contact with the wall. The edge of the chair seat should be right beneath your shoulder blades, and the yoga mat with which you covered it at the beginning should stop it from digging in too sharply. Walking your hands down the back chair legs toward the floor will increase the opening effect of the chest and heart space. If the head feels awkward, it can be supported by a cushion raised to the correct height, so the neck is still gently arched, but the head isn't hanging. If it turns out you feel you could do with an even greater backbend and stretch, release the arms, grab the elbows overhead, and hang them back (SEE ILL.42). Hold this pose for any amount of time up to ten minutes, but do come out if there is pain. Come out by bending the knees and placing the feet on the floor, and while grabbing the seat or pushing against the floor, take a big inhalation and then

raise the torso back up on the out-breath. Slide the sitting bones back on the seat and briefly, as a counterstretch, round the torso forward over the seat, resting the elbows on the backrest or thighs.

In this pose you get all the stimulating benefits of the backbend. The front of the body is stretched and with it the organs. More space is made for the lungs and thus breathing becomes fuller. The shoulders are opened and the mobility in the spine increased.

Note: This exercise is also very useful for those advanced yogis who are learning *Kapotasana* (Full Pigeon), full *Shiva Natarajasana* (Dancing Shiva, see cover photo) or other poses in which the arms need to be brought directly overhead to grab the feet. Here you would use a belt looped around the front chair legs. Lie back as described above, but bringing the arm overhead grab hold of each side of the belt with the respective hand and try walking the hands along the belt until they catch the chair leg (SEE ILL.43). As you do so, keep squeezing the elbows together. For most of us, this is everything but easy, and this version of the backbend over a chair cannot be classed as restorative.

SUPPORTED SHOULDERSTAND

(SEE ILL.44) Push that same chair a little closer to the wall and place a folded blanket and bolster on the other side. Go in

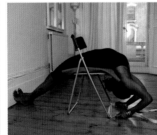

41 / 42 / 43 VARIATIONS ON BACKBEND OVER A CHAIR

sideways as you swing the legs over the seat of the chair, so its edge is in the backs of your knees and your feet are dangling off the back, toes by the wall. Now slowly lie back, bringing the shoulders onto the bolster, the back of the head on the blanket below it, and thread your arms through, as in the above exercise, past the inner front legs and grabbing the back legs with the hands. This particular action is extremely scary for many people. Though it is of course always advisable to be careful, trust that your legs and pelvis are heavier than the top of the body and thus the chair is unlikely to topple as you lie back. However, if you tense up, hold onto the chair with your hands, or panic and stop breathing, chances are that you'll injure yourself, so proceed slowly and ask someone to help you the first few times if you are afraid. Now straighten the legs up (you may need to slide them along the side, the wall being in the way), stretching the feet up so the soles, in particular the balls of the feet, are encouraged to press against the wall with the legs together. As you do this, once again you can slide the chair away a little, but be careful to remain upright with the feet in easy contact with the wall. (Taking the feet off the wall and the legs completely upright also makes for a great asana, *Viparita Karani* (inverted action, SEE ILL.45), but as this requires muscular effort, it then no longer constitutes a purely restorative pose.) It is supportive of the legwork to bind two belts around both legs, one midway up the calves and one midway up the thigh. Someone will

have to fasten the belts for you. These should be tight, though not excessively so. You may need to do a little bit of wiggling, which is not a problem providing you keep hold of the back legs of the chair. Again the edge of the chair seat may feel uncomfortable at first, but you should be able to find a position in which it does not bother your back, especially with the folded mat draped over the edge for extra padding. As with the above posture, so here the lower you walk your hands, the deeper you come into the pose. The shoulders are pulled back, the chest opens, and the chin lock is strengthened.

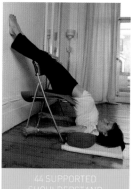

44 SUPPORTED SHOULDERSTAND

From the supported shoulderstand you will gain all the usual benefits of inverting the body, with the stilling and regulating aspect specific to *Sarvangasana*. The immune system is strengthened, venous blood flow aided, and the healthy functioning of the organs stimulated. The shoulders and chest are opened, once again stimulating fuller breathing. One learns even engagement of the legs and thus reduces imbalances in the pelvic area.

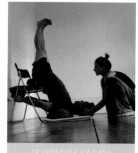

45 VIPARITA KARANI

Note: *Viparita Karani* usually refers to the legs simply being taken up the wall, often with the sacrum slightly raised by a bolster or a pile of rectangular folded blankets. This constitutes a useful alternative, especially if you haven't got an adequate chair. Remember to go in sideways, so as to be sure that the bum ends up right up against the wall. It is less powerful than Supported Shoulderstand because there is neither the full chin lock nor the opening in the shoulders and chest nor inversion of the torso, but its effect is definitely restorative and it can also be done when menstruating.

Hangovers and lack of strength due to any form of intoxication the previous day are best cured with a dynamic practice that makes you sweat, not just a restorative practice I'm afraid! Get away from guilt and the idea that you now need to punish yourself, as this only leads to injury. Treat yourself like a loving parent would: firm but nurturing. Focus on Dynamic Flow and keep building heat through *vinyasa* with *ujaii* breath and bandhas to support the capacity of your body to eliminate toxins. Stick with relatively simple movements though and don't attempt to add anything new to your repertoire of asana. Particularly if there is still alcohol or other substances sloshing around inside of you, your awareness of structure and alignment is bound not to be as sharp. On top of that, your sensitivity will be a bit dulled and you may not recognize when you are pushing into pain. At the end of the practice, give yourself plenty of time to relax and don't be surprised if you fall asleep!

YOGA NEVER LIES

If you are exhausted mentally just because you've had a dull day in the office, asana-*pranayama* will leave you feeling invigorated and alive. If, on the other hand, you feel more tired after your practice, this is a clear indication that you need to get some sleep.

MENSTRUAL PRACTICE AND THE MOON CYCLE

Some teachers hold that no yoga practice should be done during menstruation, especially not of the dynamic *vinyasa* variety. This advice is based on the fact that Hatha Yoga's main aim is to awaken kundalini, and that this is done through the harnessing and strengthening of prana *vayu*, the upward flowing of the five pranic winds. This pulling up is further supported through the application of *bandhas*, which in turn combined with *ujaii* breathing cause heat in the body, and heat as we know rises. During menstruation the body is busy ridding itself of blood and other tissues that it no longer needs. The faster and more effectively this can be done, the better. Hence at this time in the month, the downward flowing and eliminatory wind, *apana vayu*, needs to be supported. Also, the body is hot anyway during this time and thus requires cooling.

Rather than abstaining from yoga practice entirely, a slow Quantum Yoga practice, accompanied by deep nasal breathing but with a soft abdomen, will be most beneficial. As you are not "locking," avoid the jumps and any other forms of impact. Focus on Floor Work, primarily forward-bends, hip-openers, and supine poses. Some gentle backbending is also good and if the splits are practiced regularly, these are also OK. You want to avoid deep twists and anything that squashes up the abdominal region. *Bharadvajasana* is the one exception, as the twist is generated from the thoracic, not the abdominal region. Also, inversions, especially if held for a long time, must be avoided, as this can lead to endometriosis, where to put it simply, the menstrual blood flows in the wrong direction and ends up caught in the body. Therefore, don't get in the way of gravity during this time! Taking your legs up the wall in *Viparita Karani*, as described above, is a safe alternative to the inversions, as it does not tip the torso upside down.

Note: If you practice asana often and regularly, I believe that it really is a good idea to give yourself a break from it, certainly for the first two or three days of the menses. This will give the body a clear sign that you are allowing it to rest and eliminate. The result will be an increasingly regular menstrual cycle. Mine used to be all over the place; now I can practically set the clock by it. If, on the other hand, you have not yet found the discipline for consistent practice but happen to be menstruating when you do finally find the time, space, and inclination to practice, don't let that put you off! As long as you steer clear of long-held inversions, and take it a bit easier, you'll be fine to practice.

There are two great asana—*Supta Baddha Konasana* and *Upavishta Konasana*—that relieve the negative effects of menstruation, like cramping, headaches, and emotional turbulence. Hold these for a long time, so you can fully relax into them and breathe into the belly! They are also demonstrated in the accompanying DVD.

Supta Baddha Konasana, the Supine Bound Angle Pose, opens the body to receive prana and in particular makes space in the lower abdominal region, so that cramping is relieved and the blood flows freely. Have a belt, bolster, and (if you like) two sandbags handy, if you have them. Sit down on the floor, bend your knees, bring the soles of your feet together, and drop the knees to the sides. Grab the belt and loop it around the torso and inner thighs and feet, pulling it lower than the waist, so that it's on the sacrum. Be aware as you tighten it that it will tighten further as you lie back, and also position the buckle so it does not end up digging into your flesh. Lay the bolster perpendicular to your spine just behind you and lie back over it. Your arms should lay open on either side of you, with the elbows bent at right angles and in line with the shoulders, palms face up. The chin is drawn in and the neck long. If you would like to intensify the hip-opening aspect and you have no trouble with the knees, you can lay a sandbag on each inner thigh. The closer you position the sandbag to the knee, the more it will weigh the leg down. Make sure they are in the same place on each side, unless you are deliberately working on evening out an existing imbalance. *Baddha Konasana* can also be done as a forward-bend.

Note: Some people, especially those with a shorter torso, find the perpendicular bolster awkward and uncomfortable. If this is the case, place it in line and under the spine. Should the discomfort in the lower back persist, leave more of a gap between the sitting bones and bolster.

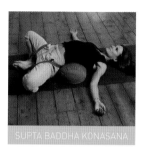
SUPTA BADDHA KONASANA

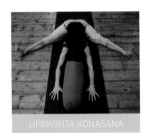
UPAVISHTA KONASANA

Upavishta Konasana is a seated forward-bend, where the legs are spread at a right angle. Engage the legs, so that knees and toes are pointing up and sit up straight. If at this stage you recognize that the spine collapses at the lumbar, sit on a block or pillow, and as with *Paschimottanasana*, spread the flesh of the sitting bones with your hands. Exhale and bend forward, reaching for the feet. As a menstrual pose, you hold *Upavishta Konasana* longer, so it is advisable to rest the head on a stack of bolsters or pillows or otherwise decreasing the height slowly as the body gives. Also, to support the work in the legs, you could lay the sandbags on the thighs near the groin. As with any forward-bend, be mindful not to hunch or tighten the shoulders. Instead, draw the shoulder blades down the back, thus expanding the heart space.

For those yogis who are very flexible in this forward-bend, it is helpful to visualize the pelvis as a basin (which it is), filled with water. Just as the water should not tip out the back, so it shouldn't tip over the front either. So, go ahead and take your chest to the floor, but once the belly flops to the ground, you know that you may have gone too far. At this stage, check the legs; chances are knees and toes are no longer facing up either. Outside the menstrual context you can use *mula* and *uddhiyana bandha* to help control this. Otherwise, make use of the props as mentioned above.

FULL AND NEW MOON DAYS

Styles such as Ashtanga Vinyasa Yoga recommend not practicing during full and new moon days, as well as on Saturdays. The reasoning behind this is that Saturn is a fiery and forceful planet and governs over Saturday, so this is the most likely day for injury. This is even more extreme on the day of the full moon, which gives excessive and erratic levels of energy. It is recommended that energy be channeled into meditation rather than asana-vinyasa practice. The new moon, on the other hand, causes a low in energy levels and rest is advisable. If one practices the same sequence daily in a strict and rigorous fashion, it makes sense to institute such days off. For male yogis this is even more important, as they are not subject to a natural cycle. However, if you truly embrace the Quantum Method, and systematically train both skill and intuition to recognize what the individual body-mind requires on the day, you no longer need to look to the moon to tell you when to rest.

QUANTUM YOGA BEFORE, AFTER AND DURING PREGNANCY

This is not a specialized book on yoga during pregnancy, so if you are about to embark on such an important part of your life, it may be advisable to purchase such a book. However, if you are an experienced yogini and have worked with the Quantum Method, you will have learned how to listen to your body and skillfully answer to its needs, which in itself is the most important aspect of pregnancy. If you allow it to, nature will guide you!

BEFORE: If you are trying to get pregnant, a generally healthy body, positive spirit, and peaceful mind will help and these are the very things that a balanced yoga practice cultivates. It is important however to realize that yoga initially promotes cleansing and letting go of the things you do not need. The *kriyas*, such as *nauli*, which is described in detail in the *Sublimatio* section of Chapter 3, especially support the body's capacity to eliminate. Also, application of *bandhas* and *ujaii* breathing promotes prana *vayu*, the upwardly directed "wind," and strengthens the body's ability to create heat, which in turn speeds up the process of purification. While you are trying to get pregnant, it may therefore be advisable to **skip** the *bandha* exercises and also soften the *ujaii*. This means that a generally more gentle and nurturing practice is a good idea!

DURING: Miscarriage is most common during the first trimester of pregnancy. This is because the fetus is not yet securely lodged in the uterus and the perfect environment for its gestation is still being built. Therefore during this time, you must be very gentle with yourself. If you have never done asana practice, I would suggest you wait until after the first three months to take up specific pregnancy yoga practice under the guidance of a qualified teacher. If, on the other hand, you are an experienced yogini, really pull the reins on any dynamic practice during this time, in the knowledge that afterwards you'll be OK to do it again.

The second trimester of pregnancy is when most of you will find that you can practice almost normally. However, as the body is releasing a softening hormone called relaxin, please do *not* push into poses. I would recommend going to about 80 percent of your capacity at this time and instead cultivating more awareness in the correct structure and alignment of each asana. In this way, pregnancy can be an extremely useful time to iron out old imbalances and heal hidden areas of weakness and restriction caused by past injury and scar tissue. It is not the time to add to your repertoire of asana.

All that was said about menstrual practice can be pretty much repeated here. All direct *bandha* exercises must be suspended. There should be no impact through jumping, and no jolting or jerky movements. Avoid deep twists, direct pressure on the abdomen, and don't overheat. I usually make space for pregnant yoginis who come to my normal Quantum Yoga classes near the window. Abdominal exercises are totally inappropriate. The belly is expanding and tightened abdominal muscles stand the risk of tearing. If you are worried about the appearance of your belly, the best thing you can do is to gently massage wheat germ or similarly vitamin E-rich oil into the skin of the abdomen. Inversions, on the other hand, can be practiced by experienced yoginis and usually offer great relief

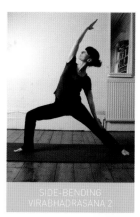

SIDE-BENDING
VIRABHADRASANA 2

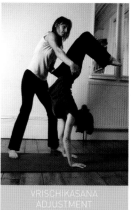

VRISCHIKASANA
ADJUSTMENT

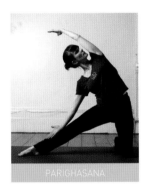

PARIGHASANA

from pressure on the ribs, particularly in the solar plexus area. For a large part of pregnancy, when you're upside down, the baby is actually the right way up! As you need to avoid falling at all costs, using the wall or having someone there to support you is advisable.

In the third and final trimester of pregnancy, your yoga practice will have to be adjusted to make room for a considerable bump and take into account the shift in weight distribution that the body needs to master. Again it is time to be really gentle on yourself. Stand and sit with your feet hip-width apart and parallel to each other. When walking, be mindful not to turn the feet out and push the belly forward as this will aggravate lower back pain. Lying on your back for any extended period is not a good idea at this time, as the the baby will otherwise weigh down on a large vein called the inferior vena cava, which carries blood back to the heart from your feet and legs. Instead, also to avoid squashing the liver, lie on the left side of your body and it often helps to place a bolster or pillow between your knees. Take plenty of rest and eat well!

LABOR: Giving birth is about allowing, not controlling. This is when Mother Nature truly knows best. You will not be able to breathe steadily through the nose as in your yoga practice and nobody expects you to smile and stay calm throughout. One of the most useful aspects of yoga while giving birth is the making of low sounds, especially the sacred primordial sound *Om*. You can channel all the pain and fear you may experience into it, and it in turn will soothe both you and the baby. Trust and embrace the wonder!

AFTER: Give yourself an adequate period of rest and time to get acquainted with the little person you have brought into this world. Note that the general recommendation is to leave six weeks after giving birth until you take up asana practice again. Don't leave too much time though, as this will make it hard to institute time for yoga into a set routine. Therefore, as soon as you are ready, start gently and just do little short practices. Don't be put off by the fact that the body feels weaker, and that the capacity to engage *mula* and *uddhiyana bandha* seems to have disappeared. All will return in due course and you are likely to be stronger for it. If you are breast-feeding, excess weight should drop off readily. Specific pelvic floor exercises are advisable. Abdominal excercises can be started once the walls have begun to pull together again. Regular Quantum Yoga practice, *vinyasa*, *bandhas*, and *ujaii* breathing will restore previous levels of fitness, flexibility, and strength. Now you have even more reason to allow the physical well-being of the body to translate into a positive and loving attitude to life.

AGE

Age is not an impediment to yoga practice. Quantum Yoga gives you the means to embrace this art at any time in your life! Allow children who join your practice to do so playfully, without holding the poses for long. The bones and tissues are still forming and you do not want to get in the way of nature. Her wisdom reigns supreme!

Unlike with many other forms of exercise, the quality of yoga increases steadily with experience. Quality is the level of awareness with which you are in the pose, and the constancy of attention you hold as you flow from one to the next. The ability to apply the attitude you cultivate in your yoga practice to all aspects of your life gives authenticity and meaning to your path. Nevertheless, even when it comes to doing fancy advanced poses, I never cease to be surprised how with advancing age my practice keeps improving. Danny Paradise said to me that you just automatically want to do it more as you get older and other distractions interest you less. Ed Clark, whose background is dance, explains that whereas dance is about the body, yoga is verily about the mind. If you can imagine it and truly believe it, it will happen. This is why one often dreams about doing an asana shortly before mastering it. I asked Clive Sheridan once what he does first thing in the morning, thinking he would enlist a disciplined regime of meditation, *pranayama*, and asana.

"I go and dig around our garden," he smiled, his bright blue eyes sparkling at me, "and then I make a cup of tea. Recently I also discovered coffee!" You could just taste how much he's been enjoying his new discovery by the guileless smile on his face. Yoga is ultimately not about what you do, but whether you do it with gratitude and remain resting in consciousness.

If one thinks of oneself as free, one is free, and if one thinks of oneself as bound, one is bound. Here this saying is true, "Thinking makes it so." Ashtavakra Gita, I, 11.

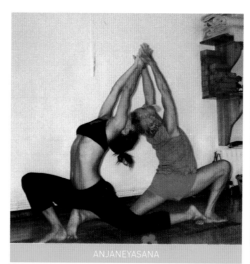

ANJANEYASANA

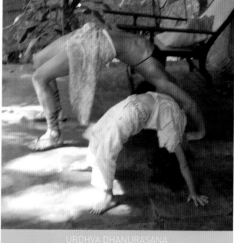

URDHVA DHANURASANA

MUDRAS AND KRIYAS

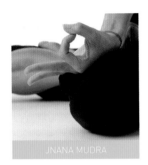

JNANA MUDRA

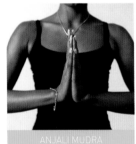

ANJALI MUDRA

MUDRAS

Mudras are usually hand gestures, like those often observed in Eastern religious icons, but some can involve other parts of or the entire body. Literally, *mudra* means "seal," and what is being sealed is an attitude or intention. Mudras fix energetic circuits and are therefore very valuable in yoga practice.

Listed below are some of the most important mudras that support asana, *pranyama*, and meditation. Some have already been explained in other chapters in the context of specific practices, and therefore appear without detailed description.

Jnana Mudra: Turn the palms up, bring the tips of the index and thumb fingers together for *jnana* mudra, which symbolizes the union of Atman and Brahman, the individual spirit realizing cosmic consciousness. The three other fingers represent the gunas, the qualities at work in the phenomenal world, that draw the mind forever back into a misidentification with conditioned existence.

Anjali Mudra: *Anjali* literally means "open palms" and denotes placing the hands in prayer. In Asia, it is used as a gesture of salutation and welcome. Yogis use it to bring the energy to the heart space. It can also be used to symbolize the higher state of union to which yogis aspire. Below is a brief excerpt from the diary I kept when studying in Mysore:

I once asked Patthabi Jois, "If you had to translate Yoga into one word only, which one would you chose?"
"Not possible! Yoga has many meanings."
He thinks. "There are five main meanings." He hesitates and then only gives one.
He raises one hand. "If this is separate," he says, and raises the other hand, on which he wears his chunky gold rings, "and this is separate,...like this is yoga." His wonderful hands are brought together in prayer position.

The following types of mudras are discussed in other sections:

Vishnu Mudra (see *Pure Pranayama*, earlier in this chapter)
Yoni Mudra (see *Pure Pranayama*, earlier in this chapter)
Kechari Mudra (see *Subtle Anatomy*, Chapter 2)
Shambhavi Mudra (see *Meditation*, Chapter 3)

KRIYAS

Cleanliness, or *saucha*, is one of the Niyamas (second Limb of Yoga) listed by Patanjali and is as important today as it was when the Sutras were composed. As already mentioned in Chapter One in the *Important Scriptures* section, the Hatha Yoga Pradipika enumerates six major cleansing actions, referred to as the *Shat Karma Kriya*. These are listed below, but due to the probably deliberately obscure nature of some of these practices, I will only go into detail with those that

I actually advocate and practice. On waking in the morning (*kapha* time), it is important to cleanse the nose, throat, mouth, and chest, which are the *kapha*, or mucus, regions of the body. Those individuals with a *kapha prakriti* (constitution) will find they produce more *kapha* in the morning than a *vata* or *pitta prakriti* individual, and need to take care to expel it.

1. *Dhauti* means "to wash." This refers to internal and external washing and can be done with air, water, gauze, turmeric, and even the beat stem of a banana tree. The rectum, bowels, tongue, ears, eyes, sinuses, and throat are all kept clean through varying ways. I assume that most yogis reading this book brush their teeth regularly and floss. Tongue-scraping is a good idea, but not excessively. The same can be said for using ear-buds or cotton swabs, which should be kept to a minimum. I also advocate the Asian way of using water to clean one's bottom post-evacuation, and personally I love the French idea of the bidet.

Agni sari is included in the *dhautis*, and I have already described this practice in the *Sublimatio* section of Chapter 3. It is useful in strengthening the inner flame and thus the body's general capacity to assimilate and eliminate.

2. *Basti* is the equivalent of an enema, and the Hatha Yoga Pradipika describes it as a process done with water or air. Colonic irrigation with water (often containing Ayurvedic herbs) can be very useful in regulating a person's digestion that has become sluggish through the accumulation of toxins or bad eating habits. However, as with all things, I recommend measure. Some people make colonic irrigation into a dietary habit, with view of keeping their weight down. This can easily backfire, as digestion will become lazy, and also too many healthy bacteria and minerals are washed out.

3. *Neti* is primarily designed to treat phlegm and is done using water, thread, milk, and ghee. I personally stick with lightly salted and filtered lukewarm water, and use a *neti* pot to pour it up one nostril and out the other. *Neti*, too, can be overdone and I think once or twice a week suffices. Remember to tip your head slightly to the side and forward and of course breathe through the *mouth*!

4. *Trataka*, or "fixing your gaze," can be done internally (eyes closed) or externally. For the latter often the flame of a candle is used. Try to stop your eyes from blinking and welcome the tears. As the eyes water, they are being cleansed in the most natural way possible, from the inside out.

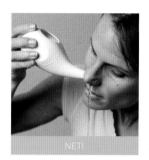

NETI

5. *Nauli*, or the "churning" of the abdomen, is already described in Sublimatio (Chapter 3). It has three parts, left, right, and center. It is easiest first thing in the morning on an empty stomach.

6. *Kapalabhati*, or "shining skull," is already described in the Pranayama section. The fact that it is listed as a *kriya* indicates just how powerful this "bouncing" of the diaphragm through short, sharp exhalations is in eliminating any residual air that is not being exchanged by the tidal breath. There are also exercises of pulling water in through the nose and out through the mouth and vice-versa that are referred to as *kapalabhati* in the Hatha Yoga Pradipika.

Saucha, of course, also refers to the purity of your actions and thoughts. Keeping the body and your immediate environment clean does tend to support clarity of mind and inspire clear behavior and lucid speech. However, just because a person's appearance may not be clean, they should not be judged, as saints come in many disguises. Equally, even the most spotless prophet may well be covering up dirty deeds and impure intentions. Actions still always speak louder than words or appearance.

SOUND, VISION AND TOUCH: FURTHER SUPPORTS FOR QUANTUM YOGA PRACTICE

NADA: THE ART OF LISTENING

Nada Yoga, the yoga of sound and music, originated around 200 BCE, but had its roots in the Vedic *Shabda* Yoga, shabda being the primordial sound. The *nada* is the resonance of the divine in our body-mind. It is the root vibration that runs through the entire fabric of reality. To hear it we must still the chatter of the mind.

In Nada Yoga, it is the heart that listens. The name of the heart chakra, *anahata* chakra, is related to the concept of *anahata nada*, the "unstruck" sound. It is a sound that is not caused by anything, that springs out of itself. Its eternal resonance can only be heard when there is no motive, no imposition of what the ego wants to hear, nor what the mind, based on memory and inference, construes it should be hearing. Pure listening is interested only in capturing what is really there. Yet the primordial sound is elusive and very difficult to pierce through to. Therefore, we can use *ahata nada*, or "struck" audible sound, to hold our attention and encourage us to listen out for even more subtle universal vibrations. Natural sound and music made with pure intention and skill represent such captivating sound.

In the hierarchy of the senses, hearing is regarded as the most refined. The aim is to ultimately control the senses at will (*pratyahara*; fifth Limb of Yoga), withdrawing them from their objects to turn the attention inward. Many Hatha Yoga traditions would argue that the use of music to accompany asana practice could represent a distraction from the breath and cause further mental turbulence. When it comes to establishing a personal practice however, until the capacity for total concentration (dharana, sixth Limb of Yoga) has been established, the senses can be of use in supporting focus. For example, refining one's hearing with the use of subtle natural sound, sacred chants or hymns, and gentle, rhythmic, or uplifting music will lead to a greater capacity to pay attention to the gentle waves of your inner song. Sound support in the form of music can be very useful in ensuring an unbroken stream of consciousness, particularly in the context of the consistency of rhythm that *vinyasa* requires to cultivate an even flow of breath, movement, and effort.

Repeated chanting of mantras is also very effective in getting beyond the mind (*man-* refers to the "mind", *-tra* implies "transcend", "liberate" or "instrument"). This practice is referred to as *japa* and uses a beaded rosary, or mala, to further hold the practitioner's attention. The sacred Sanskrit syllables that make up mantras lend themselves particularly well to such chanting. Even if the content is not understood, their vibration is said to carry transformative powers. *Aum* represents the root vibration. Manifestation began with a movement of subatomic particles that caused sound and chanting *Aum* is the closest we can get to reproducing this sound. It is like returning to the source of existence itself. It is the beginning (*A* for Brahma, the Creator), being (*U* for Vishnu, the Sustainer), and dissolution (*M* for Shiva, the Destroyer) all in one and is therefore timeless and eternal. *Aum* is what some cultures would refer to as God.

The use of the sense of sight in establishing one-pointed focus through *drishti* or such cleansing practices as *trataka* serve to demonstrate ultimately the same dichotomy that runs through all spiritual practice. As the focus sharpens and there is total uncompromised attention, the gaze actually softens and loses its sharpness, which leads to a blurring and ultimate dissolution of the object one had focused on. This soft focus echoes the attitude of the mind in a state of absorption (dhyana, seventh Limb of Yoga).

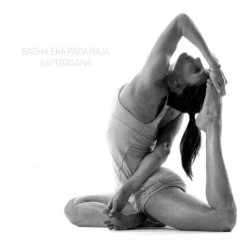

BADHA EKA PADA RAJA
KAPOTASANA

The ultimate limb of yoga, or *samadhi*, represents a state that is beyond the duality of perceiver and perceived. Thus it is without describable characteristics, but as it represents the total emancipation from the control of the senses, ultimate freedom from the activities of the mind, the closest one can describe it is as being of the nature of bliss (*ananda*). It is unlike conventional happiness in that it is without an opposite or condition, it has no beginning or end, and pertains to no one in particular, but it is (*sat*) and it can be realized (*cit*)—Sat-cit-ananda: being-knowing-bliss.

THEME, INSPIRATION, CREATIVITY

Even more effective than setting an intention for one's practice is to choose a theme. This theme may be based on a spiritual concept you have been contemplating, an aspect of nature, or even just a poetic reference or artistic inspiration. Often the theme will be informed by the peak posture or postures you have chosen. The peak posture forms the apex of your sequence. Thus all preceding asana prepare for this challenge, and those following it consolidate the accumulated energy and establish a lasting state of inner serenity and ease. For instance, if your peak posture is *Eka Pada Raja Kapotasana* (One-legged King Pigeon) from the advanced Birds Sequence, your theme is that of freedom, true lightness that can only be the result of a firm connection to Mother Earth. You should prepare this beautiful asana through hip- and shoulder-openers, backbends, and core-strengthening exercises.

I would like to discuss here the significance of the Sanskrit names of asana. Not only do they provide you with inspiration and often awaken an interest for further study, more importantly they provide an insight into the essence of a pose. One of the reasons I chose the King Pigeon as the peak pose for the Birds Sequence and put its photo on the cover of the first Quantum Healing Sounds CD is because the pigeon was a posture I struggled with greatly. In fact, I got seriously injured while being adjusted in *Kapotasana*, when a vertebra slid out of my spine. I realized that I needed to understand this asana and form a bond with the animal it was named after, undesireable, filthy urban birds that they are treated as. There was some sort of message here. I sat at Trafalgar Square and watched the pigeons, particularly the one that was missing a leg. It stood out, because it was white, more like a dove. To balance, it seemed to have pulled its body mass upward in the most spectacular manner, wobbling along quite regally in a broad swagger, with its chest sticking out and beak up in the air. I realized then that *Eka Pada Raja Kapotasana* was primarily about puffing up the chest and stabilizing the rather awkward foundation of the pose by widening it. To safeguard the back, one had to pull away from the earth through mula bandha, and draw the navel down and drop the tailbone

with *uddhiyana bandha*, reducing the bend in the lumbar and directing it into the thoracic spine. My attention previously had been only in the back, but as soon as I brought it also to the heart space at the front, I understood the pose. With it came a message from my little friend, namely that the seemingly

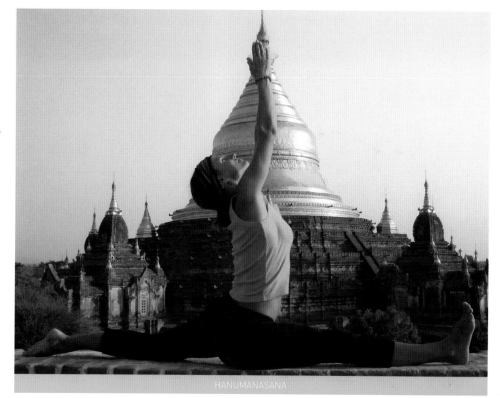

HANUMANASANA

impossible mission of the urban yogi to find peace amidst the chaos could only ever result from embracing and learning to love it.

Many of the asana names also refer to stories from the Ramayana and Mahabharata or other sacred scriptures, as well as being named after the sages that composed them. These may inspire the yogi in creating their sequence, as well as reveal key aspects of the pose. For example, *Hanumanasana*, the front splits, is named after one of the heroes of the Ramayana, Hanuman, the monkey god. This courageous warrior took one giant stride from India to Sri Lanka to save the virtue of Sita, Rama's wife, who had been abducted by an evil demon. Indeed, it does take courage, skill, and perseverance to master this challenging posture. Many an impatient yogi has been injured in it (including myself). This can be avoided if the posture is truly understood as a

stride, not simply a stretch with a downward release into gravity. In fact the contrary is the case. There should be a true effort to keep the hips squared up, by digging the heel of the flexed front foot into the ground, thus "sucking" the leg back into the pelvis, and keeping the back foot's toes tucked under and the knee off the floor. *Bandha triyam* needs to be fully established to safeguard the lumbar region and check the goal-orientated ego-mind that just wants to go down. Hanuman would have ended up in the sea had he not been fully attentive to where he was heading while skillfully using his firm connection to the land he came from to ensure forward motion. Hanumanasana should be practiced in this way until the muscles are so open that the legs are on the ground, while the hips remain squared. Only then is one truly ready to release the back foot toes, lift the arms overhead and perhaps even go into variations of the back leg, such as Pigeon or Frog.

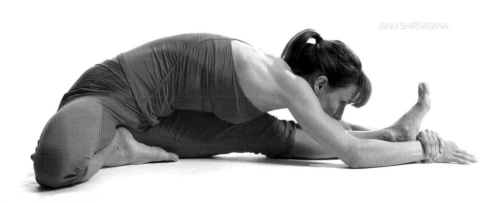
JANU SHIRSASANA

Even the asana names that simply make reference to the physics or geometry of the pose, such as the Triangle or any name that includes the term *kona*, linguistically related to the English "corner" and denoting a right angle of sorts, will set a clear parameter for the asana's execution. Sometimes, such as in the case of the seated one-legged forward-bend *Janu Shirsasana*, what the name suggests is less straightforward. Janu means knee and shirsa means head. If this means that we are encouraged to bring our head to the straight-leg knee, we would have to be deliberately rounding our back and some styles actually do. One could argue however that reference is actually being made here to the head of the bent-leg knee, which points in varying directions depending on what version of the pose, A, B, or C, one has chosen.

On a final note in our discussion of asana names, it should of course be mentioned that Sanskrit is regarded as a sacred language, containing the purest of sound vibrations. Therefore, knowing a name of an asana with its correct pronunciation may inspire yoga practice just through the beauty of its sound. Furthermore, from a practical point of view, knowing the original asana names means that you can communicate a posture to a fellow yogi even if they don't speak your language. Be aware, though, that an impediment to such a universal understanding of asana is the fact that even in India varying yoga traditions call the same posture by different names.

YANTRA AND MANDALA

Music is not the only artistic medium that has been used to great effect in supporting meditation and yoga practice. Yantra and mandala use the visual medium to create cosmic diagrams in which the mind can center and eventually get beyond itself. The yantra is the simpler of the two.

Yantras represent tools for meditation, *yantra* meaning "support" or "instrument." *Mandala* means "circle" or "completion" and meditations on mandalas are usually more complex, involving contemplation on various symbolic meanings associated with different regions of the mandala. Both represent microcosmic pictures of the macrocosm of the universe and play on the idea that in its archetypal shapes and colors the universe reflects itself. The human eye recognizes these and is drawn to their simplicity, which overrides the personalized trivia that usually occupies the mind.

Yantras are black and white, whereas a mandala can be very colorful. The simple shapes of yantras are said to emit very specific frequencies, which resonate with the mind, resulting in a communion with a certain sphere of universal energy. Where forms interpenetrate, the dynamic interaction of correspondent energies can result in potent visual receptacles for mental focus. Both yantras and mandalas are symmetrical in shape and thus draw the eye to the core of the diagram, at the center of which we find the dot, or *bindu*. These charts are based on Hindu cosmology, which describes the earth through a four-cornered square dilineated by the horizon's relationship with the sunrise and sunset, the north and south directions. Mandalas play an important role in Vedic astrology, as well as in Vastu Shastra, the Vedic teachings on correct town, architectural, and interior planning in harmony with the directional forces.

In the practice of asana in Quantum Yoga, the body itself is regarded as a microcosm and used as an object for meditation. Here, too, geometric shapes are used to align the flow of energy and challenge the body to return to its innate state of balance.

LOTUS MANDALA: The vajra, the diamond thunderbolt at its center, symbolizes the ascent of the body- mind away from disease and delusion towards grace and enlightenment.

QUANTUM YANTRA: This yantra was designed to represent a state of balance between the doshas in the microcosm of the human body-mind.

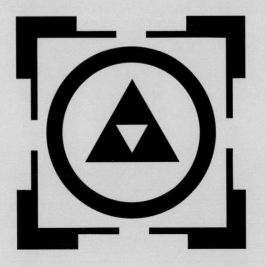

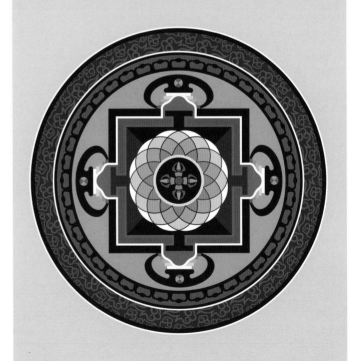

Listed below are shapes commonly found in yantras and mandalas.

The **SHATKONA** is a six-pointed star representing the union of Shiva and Shakti, *purusha* and *prakriti*. It is symbolic of the sacred union of opposite energies, and also the perfect meditative balance achieved between humanity and God.

The **CIRCLE**, or chakra, symbolizes rotation, spiraling energy, and the evolution of the macrocosm. It also represents perfection, bliss, and the void. Its element is air, relating to the *vata dosha*.

The **DOT**, or *bindu*, symbolizes Shiva consciousness in tantric iconography.

The **TRIANGLE**, *trikona*, represents Shakti energy.
The **DOWNWARD-POINTING TRIANGLE**, or *yoni*, symbolizes the feminine aspect in nature.
The **UPWARD-POINTING TRIANGLE** represents *agni* fire and symbolzies spiritual aspiration.

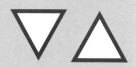

The **SQUARE**, *bhupura*, represents earth (*prthivi*). The outer square is to the bindu what earth is to ether, a movement from gross to subtle.

The **LOTUS**, or *padma*, represents the pure mind and the state of emancipation from the "mud" of the phenomenal world.

CREATING YOUR IDEAL YOGA PRACTICE: GETTING STARTED

Creation requires us to overcome the initial resistance we all feel to change. I am very familiar with that time-waster called procrastination. Why, since I've started this book, I must have rearranged my wardrobe at least five times, had endless meaningful chats with the lovely lady who makes my take-away coffees, and for the first time ever established an impeccable order in my bookshelves, all in order to get away from the actuality of what I really set out to do—write this book. Giving birth to anything new, especially when we really care about it, brings with it an army of resistance, and can be a very painful process indeed. How then can you cultivate the initiative, confidence, and enthusiasm to start designing and doing your ideal yoga practice?

Once I had fully recognized that I'd be better off with an individualized and varying Quantum practice, it still took me a long time to make spontaneous, intelligent, and joyful creation in yoga a regular occurrence. I'd hesitantly step onto the mat, having decided: Today I will really tune in and see what comes up. Nothing much would come up, except thoughts pertaining to what else I could be doing with my time. So I would either punish myself by rigorously defaulting to a well-known sequence, or give up and furiously do something else, knowing full well that I'd let myself down. When I had injuries, I would design a whole set of restorative exercises, but hardly ever get around to doing them. Also there always

were difficult poses I yearned to master, but I didn't know how to approach them if they were not part of the sequences I knew by heart.

The first step in changing this pattern was to set myself a time when I would start the practice and fix how long I would spend. This became a sacred time for that day, which, no matter what was happening around me, I would spend on the mat. With regards to the yoga mat, I do sometimes practice without it, but I find that in the encounter of inner resistance it is useful to demarcate a sacred space. There would be days that I would struggle with such fierce demons that I would end up a shaking wreck huddled on my mat. However, I would not leave and the longer I sat with these self-denying thoughts and worked with this body that seemed totally unwilling to cooperate, the more constructive this conversation with myself became. Ultimately, I believe that these seemingly "futile" times are just as useful as days when the practice flows magically. It is just another form of sadhana, and when it comes to spiritual practice, as long as you approach it with an earnest and fervent heart, you are opening to grace.

There are ways though that you can avoid this kind of creative paralysis:

1) Start gently! Remember that Sublimatio is when you are feeling your way into your body. Cultivate "beginner's mind." Allow yourself to be childlike, innocently exploring your being as though for the very first time. In this way you avoid preconceived notions of what you could or should be like and take yourself into the here and now. *Santosha*, one of Patanjali's *niyamas*, is often translated as "contentment," but to me it indicates being with what is really there rather than projecting.

2) Assess what part of your being needs the most attention! Quantum Yoga offers the science of the Ayurvedic *doshas* as a useful aid in self-healing. Do remember that the three doshas coexist and very often it is not entirely clear which one requires regulating. Nevertheless, this system is a great aid in identifying what the overall flavor or tone of your practice should be.

Vata: If this *dosha* predominates, you require grounding. You are feeling unstable, flighty, impulsive, and dry, as though the state of warm and powerful stillness from which you originated is but a remote memory.

Pitta: You need to chill out and cool down. In the midst of being preoccupied with what needs to get done and how you will go about doing it, you have forgotten to actually experience the moment. You find it hard to be receptive or contain feelings that alternate between anger and joy, which leaves you feeling exhausted.

Kapha: You feel heavy and find it hard to gather the momentum to actually do something about it. When laziness overcomes you, there is a general sense of stagnation that leads to inertia, toxicity, and lack of enthusiasm.

Respond openly to the impulses you get while flowing through your practice. Asana-*pranayama* are such powerful tools to self-discovery that you may find you have to adjust your focus somewhat as you go along in order to maximize the benefits of that particular session. Nevertheless, beware of the mind's trickery and do not end the practice prematurely unless there is a real risk of injury or an emergency you need to attend to.

3) Pick a theme! What inspires you today? Is there a peak pose you would like to work towards? Would you like to dedicate your practice to someone, an animal, a plant, an idea? Is there a certain flavor, color, sentiment, or image you feel would be useful to take yourself back to if the monkey-mind wanders? Setting a theme gives you a thread, and although you can be flexible and allow little subplots to form in the story of your practice, you always come back to that central theme and in this way integrate all parts into a coherent whole.

4) Play music! If you feel this will support your practice, choose some inspiring tunes to play. Again select it in accordance with what kind of charge you would like to give your practice. Don't make an empty habit of this, though. Many times it may be more appropriate to practice in silence. If you have the luxury of being outdoors in nature, the resonance of natural sounds can also have very beneficial effects.

5) Be structured! Use the Quantum Grouping and Sequencing laws to systematically carry out a balanced sequence. Intuition and creativity are far more powerful when they are placed in a logical framework that has been prepared through years of research and derives from empirical knowledge as a result of trial and error.

Do not linger too long in any one group. I have provided suggested percentages of the time to spend depending on what *dosha* you are regulating. Naturally these are only vague indications, as you may be preparing the body-mind for a peak posture for which a particularly inflexible or weak part of your body may need to be released or strengthened. Nevertheless, remember that all groupings will contain asana that allow you to work into these areas. For example, if preparation for deep backbending is what you require, it won't just be in the Backbends section that you will find what you need. The body-mind must be approached holistically. The reason that you cannot do *Eka Pada Raja Kapotasana* (the One-Legged King Pigeon) for instance may not be lack of flexibility in the back, but where you are bending it from, as well as the hips providing a stable foundation, the shoulders and arm muscles stretching and the heart space opening. All parts of the body must be in accord. This coherence extends to the breath, the intention, and the state of mind from which the thought of celebrating this asana emerged. A deep understanding of structure and alignment, the energetic direction, as well as the observation of nature and philosophical underpinnings of that particular asana will all contribute to its mastery. Ultimate mastery is a merging with the asana, the moment when you are no longer practicing it, but you have fully surrendered to its sacred geometry and aligned yourself with the elemental aspect of reality it reveals. It becomes you, and that is yoga—union.

6) Don't be distracted! What are your priorities? If you view yoga practice simply as me-time, the moment the going gets tough and you are struggling through and hating every bit of it, it suddenly won't feel like me-time anymore and will quickly be replace by another fad. Yoga is not pampering. Regarding as "me-time" a path that leads to the temporary dissolution of the idea of self and a realization of the absolute or divine self is a contradiction in terms. Yoga will be arduous and you will encounter pain and resistance that will be nothing short of unpleasant. It is therefore much more useful to be clear from the outset that yoga is a commitment to truth. Unpeeling layers and layers of conditioning from your sublime essence will require dedication, skill, faith, discipline, curiosity, and a will to live life to its fullest.

7) Don't set yourself up for failure! If your goals are realistic, you may be pleasantly surprised. Remember again that the quality of your practice should not be judged by how fancy a set of asana you can perform, but by the level of awareness with which you practice. Often the capacity to fully realize the subtle effects of the simpler asana requires a higher level of concentration and a truly refined approach.

8) Regular moderate practice is more effective than rare intense bouts. Your body-mind will respond far more favorably to short but regular quality time dedicated to spiritual practice, than infrequent punishing sessions that leave you aching for days. If half an hour is all you can manage, Quantum Yoga provides you with the possibility of a short but balanced and effective practice. It should be noted here though that times of intense immersion, such as going on retreat or just taking a few days off to reconnect, form an important part of most yogis' paths. If these times complement an otherwise relatively balanced life, you will have found the best way.

9) Begin by learning the Basic Quantum Sequences and practicing them in alternation, choosing to regulate the dosha you know to be most pervasive in your type and present condition. This will constitute a fully balanced practice. Then introduce variations from other yoga styles, exercise routines, or spiritual disciplines you know to be beneficial.

Alternatively, simply explore the possibility of constructing a sequence from different parts of the three Basic Quantum Sequences (Birds, Heroes, Lotus Mandala), all the while adhering to the Grouping and Sequencing Laws. Finally, sit down, and using the form on the next page, write your own sequence. Refine it with use. Eventually, spontaneous creation during the practice will become possible, but just like any other craft, for the best results, you must hone your skill slowly and patiently.

10) Aim high! I know this advice seems to contradict point 7, so allow me to explain what I mean by setting high standards. In my many years of teaching, I have observed that most people, particularly in the so-called West, tend to shortchange themselves. We come from a culture that celebrates individuality, financial wealth, and physical beauty as the ultimate achievements. Yet none of these things pertain to our inner well-being, or furthermore to the true spiritual potential that is the same for everyone. To some it may sound radical that I practice because I am after enlightenment in this lifetime, that my aim is to be completely free from fear and permanently in touch with the existential bliss that the entire manifest world emanates from. How dare a person be so arrogant as to believe that we can access a level of consciousness that is beyond the ordinary? And that furthermore, to think that every time we do so, we have set another milestone towards not only personal liberation, but universal peace and harmony? How could anyone possibly think that what we do matters so much!

I know that every breath ever taken matters enormously and that in this intricate web we call our world, grace holds out her open palms at all times to catch anyone who turns to her. Our lives may seem insignificant in comparison with the enormity of the universe, but is it not our awareness of that very universe that imbues it with relevance? Size becomes insignificant as we enter the realm of pure consciousness that transcends all limitations of time and space. Therefore, I humbly challenge you, my dear reader, to entertain the possibility of freedom from the cage the mind can and will put you in if you allow it to. May our spirits meet instead in that infinite sanctuary of stillness and joy to which all yoga practice ultimately and invariably leads.

QUANTUM YOGA SEQUENCE PLANNER

TITLE	
THEME	
PEAK POSE	
MAIN DOSHA TO BE REGULATED (IF ANY)	
ESTIMATED TOTAL TIME OF SEQUENCE	
INJURIES/AREAS THAT REQUIRE ATTENTION	

Please choose music and prepare props that you may need before you commence the practice!

1) SUBLIMATIO

2) DYNAMIC FLOW

3) STANDING POSES

4) STANDING & ARM BALANCES

5) FLOOR WORK

6) ABDOMINALS

7) BACKBENDS

8) INVERSIONS

9) RELAXATION

10) MEDITATION

LARA'S YOGA BIOGRAPHY

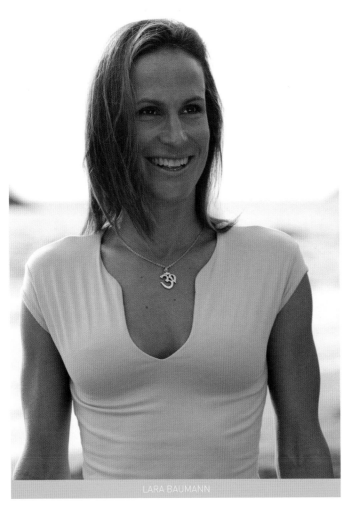
LARA BAUMANN

My first encounter with yoga came at an early age, growing up in Madras as the daughter of a diplomat father. After a long period of illness, my mother decided to take up yoga practice on the advice of a friend. She soon lost interest however, and her personal yoga teacher was relegated to teaching the children. When I rediscovered yoga practice twenty years later, memories of my early experience surfaced and it seemed like the most natural way of working with the body.

Initially my adult study of yoga was mostly academic, part of a Master's Degree in Religious Studies I completed at the School of Oriental and African Studies (University of London) and my tutoring of Comparative Religions in Oxford. My interest at that time was primarily in Buddhist meditation. Thus it was at a ten-day silent retreat in southern Thailand that I actually got "hooked" on asana practice, by a newly qualified Shivananda teacher who had volunteered to relieve us of our aching backs with optional early morning yoga sessions. It was a blessing to have the opportunity, with a beginner's mind and an untrained body, to experience the initial effects of physical yoga practice within the context of daily meditation and ten days of silence. Not only was there greater ease and an immediate increase in comfort, but I could very clearly perceive that a total energetic realignment had been initiated in my body. The breath, which had previously simply been an object of focus to support concentration, now became a measure of my depth of consciousness. I started perceiving it as an indicator of a fine inner balance and an eternal connection to the essence of all things. As my body transformed into a more steady and receptive container for prana, the vital life force taken in through the breath, the heart softened and the mind more often gave in to stillness.

Upon my return to London, I joined weekly Iyengar classes that took place in an underheated classroom in a Notting Hill backyard. It was the only yoga class I could find in this part of town in the mid-nineties. How things have changed! I discovered Ashtanga Vinyasa with a cover teacher who defiantly introduced a few Sun Salutations into the otherwise static class, and then my love for yoga reached another level. An injury at a party where I cut my leg meant I had to take up restorative practice, which only served to reinforce my dedication to the path. I also discovered Shadow Yoga, which served as a counterbalance to the somewhat forced exaltation that Ashtanga left me with. Shadow practice was more grounding and strengthening, but nowhere near as uplifting for the spirits and as opening as the Ashtanga. So I practiced the two for a while. Usually in the evening, while relaxing and listening to music, I would spontaneously start flowing into a free practice and often feel afterwards like I'd worked more deeply, honestly, and lovingly than in my more formal

morning practices. Why couldn't I always tune in like that, creating spontaneously and intuitively knowing what I needed? Yet, having been trained in disciplines that perpetuate the belief that one must adhere to fixed sequences, because "that is the system," I was reluctant to stray and felt like a rebel when I did. At other times, I simply did not feel inspired or confident enough to create and thus would default back to the familiar. Soon I realized that I would not receive the full benefits of yoga until I had found a way to integrate what I had learned into a coherent personal practice. Out of this mission, Quantum Yoga was born.

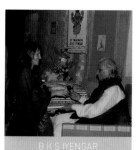

B K S IYENGAR

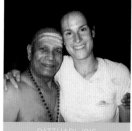

PATTHABI JOIS

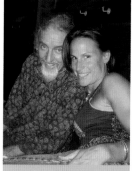

CLIVE SHERIDAN

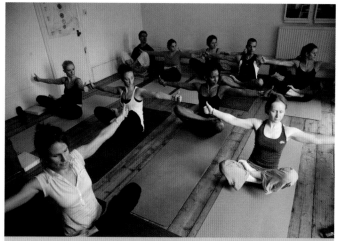

OMSTATION3 APPRENTICESHIP CLASS 07 / 08

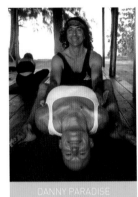

DANNY PARADISE

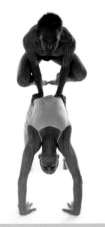

EDWARD CLARK

In my years as an apprentice, I traveled to study with Patthabi Jois and his grandson Sharath in Mysore and was invited to Pune to learn from B. K. S. Iyengar and his children Gita and Prashant. These were interesting experiences that to me only highlighted the fact that yoga is a very personal path and cannot be pinned down to a single style or creed. I finally found a true teacher in Clive Sheridan, who encouraged me to integrate regular pranayama and more seated meditation into my daily asana practice. Clive taught classic Indian poses and varying *Suryanamaskara* (Sun Salutations), which inspired me to start weaving additional poses into my sequences and generally broadening my alphabet of asana. I was also fortunate enough to take up Ashtanga again with Danny Paradise, whose light-hearted approach and open-minded outlook was unlike the rigidity and competitiveness that I had experienced before. Danny's interest in shamanism and his deep love of nature seemed to give back authenticity to this style of yoga. OmStation3, my yoga studio in Notting Hill Gate, was awarded the Yoga Alliance certification in 2004 and I took on my first twelve apprentices in that year. In spring 2005, I did my own formal teacher training with Sharon Gannon and David Life at Jivamukti Yoga in upstate New York. In the past years, I have been practicing with Edward Clark (founder of Tripsichore, a yoga theatre company), and my asana practice, as well as the use of breath and my understanding of the laws of physics, has literally developed in leaps and bounds.

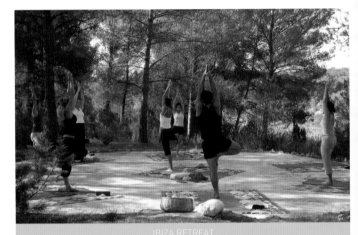

IBIZA RETREAT

GOA RETREAT

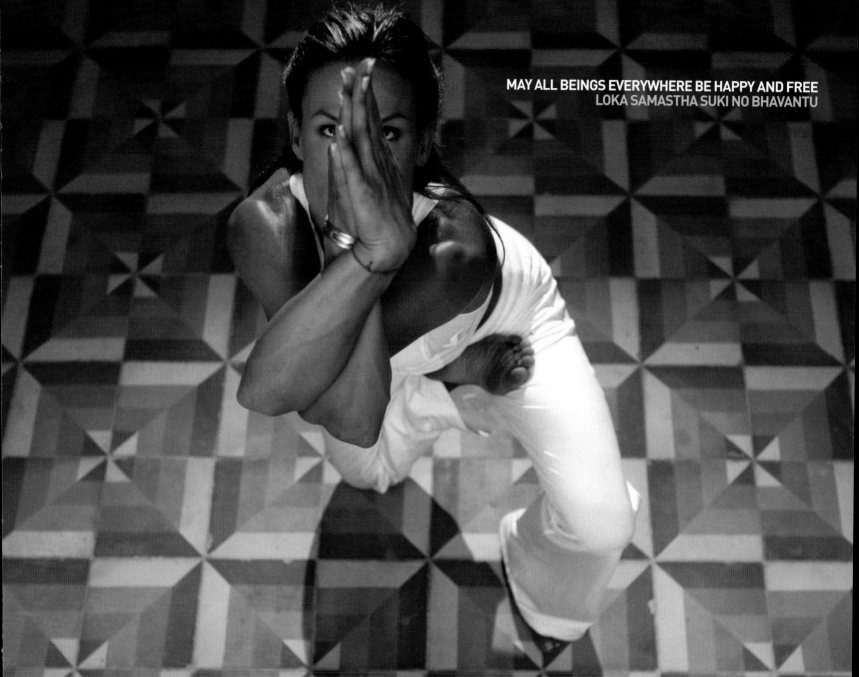

MAY ALL BEINGS EVERYWHERE BE HAPPY AND FREE
LOKA SAMASTHA SUKI NO BHAVANTU

ACKNOWLEDGEMENTS

Thank you first of all to my apprentices and students, for you have been my greatest teachers. The OmStation3 teaching team without whose support I could not have kept the studio going whilst writing, recording and filming. My mother, who's just always there for me; you're the best! Patrick Shlash, whose "Coaching I-Ching" reliably brings clarity when there is confusion. Dr Matthew Clark whose advice on all things Sanskrit has been invaluable. Arjuna van der Kooij who found one of my articles on the internet, put me in touch with Mandala Publishing and became the editor of this book. Nic Hinton without whose design talent and stamina the Quantum project may well have crash-landed in its final phase. Jean-Philippe Woodland who is responsible for most of the photos in this book, often taken under enormous time, space, light and financial restraints. Claire Russell for her beautiful illustrations. Celine Bruckner for her ideas and competent support. Hayley Johns for helping with the edit. Robin Pender for the blood, sweat and tears that went into making the Quantum Yoga DVD.

All musicians, producers, and mastering specialists who have provided musical accompaniment for the DVD, often from the previously released Quantum Yoga CD's. Clare Lorimer for her advice on patenting. Ann -Louise Holland, Mel Enright and Lainey Young for sharing your skills in promotion. Chloe Ansell for being my trusted assistant. Neera Vasisht for generously sharing her knowledge of Ayurveda. Gary Derrick, my osteopath, for his incredible understanding of the human body and effective suggestions on restorative exercise. My brother Joel for helping me out when I have another computer crisis. Jonathan Monjack for patient legal advice. And of course all the rest of my fabulous family and friends for the love, fun and times we share!

Photography ©Jean-Philippe Woodland 2008
www.jphwoodland.com

FOOTNOTES

1. David Frawley. "The Aryan-Dravidian Controversy." The Hindu Universe. HinduNet Inc. www.hindunet.org/hindu_history/ancient/aryan/aryan_frawley_1.html

2. Indra Devi, Hinduism Today. www.hinduismtoday.com. www.hinduismtoday.com/archives/2002/10-12/52-54_indradevi.shtml

3. Amit Goswami, PhD, in *What the Bleep Do We Know!?* (motion picture). William Arntz, Betsy Chasse, Mark Vicente (directors & producers). (2004) Los Angeles: Twentieth Century Fox.

4. Stephen Linsteadt, "Quantum Physics and Holographic Repatterning" Natural Healing House™. www.naturalhealinghouse.com/quantumhr.htm

5. Ken Wilber, *Quantum Questions* (Boston, Shambhala, 2001), p.83.

6. Trademark, Mister Booja Booja organic vegan chocolates.

7. Ken Wilber (editor), Quantum Questions (Boston: Shambala, 1984, 2001), 8.

8. Arthur Eddington, ibid. 196–197.

9. All Ayurveda charts were kindly composed by Neera Vashisht.

10. Reference: *Ashtanga Hridaya*, *Suthrasthana*, Chapter 1, sloka 8.

11. Reference: Ashtanga Samgraha, Suthrasthana, Chapter 21, sloka 8.

12. Edward F. Edinger, Anatomy of the Psyche (Illinois, Open Court Publishing, 1994), 117.

13. Ibid Quantum Physics chapter. Stephen Linsteadt.

14. Donna Farhi has investigated this phenomenon further. See her articles such as "Coming Together: The Sacroiliac Joint". Handout at Triyoga Teacher's workshop London, 2005.

15. I do a few of my own interpretations of these on the Quantum Master Sequence DVD "Capricious Shiva", which will be released before the end of 2008. If you would like to learn more, I would strongly recommend Ed Clark's challenging DVD, *Tripsichore Yoga*.

16. The three Advanced Quantum Sequences Infinity Trees, Beauty and Leaping Salmon, have yet to be publisized. Any new publication will appear on www.quantumyoga.co.uk.

GLOSSARY

Advaita "nondual", traditions that regard Brahman as the sole reality, that we are already part of. Enlightenment is achieved by realising this

Amrit the sacred nectar of immortality, which drops form the bindu

Asana "seat", most often translated as "posture" or "pose". It is the third of the eight-limbs of yoga

Atman individual soul or spirit

Ayurveda the "science of life". Knowledge pertaining to the maintenance of a person's ideal way of life, which embraces a holistic approach to health, honouring individual body-mind types

Bandha Triyam gripping of the three main locks simultaneously

Bandhas "locks," subtle internal muscular grips or holds, such as mula bandha, the root lock at the perineum, Uddhiyana Bandha, the abdominal lock, and Jalandhara Bandha, or the chin lock. Bandhas can also refer to firm connections to the outer world such as Hasta, hand and Pada Bandha, foot lock.

Bhagavad Gita "Song of the Lord" was recorded in the epic Mahabharata (eighth to sixth century BCE), and tells the story of Arjuna, a kshatriya, or warrior prince, who in a moment of doubt refuses to fight. Upon which his charioteer Krishna, an avatar, or incarnation, of Vishnu reveals to him in a great discourse the quintessential secrets of yoga

Bhakti Yoga the deliverance through grace that results from devotion

Bhoga enjoyment of life

Bija mantra root sound

Bindu "point", located in the head at the posterior fontanel near the pineal gland and represents the void from whence we became manifest

Brahma "the creator" god, who together with Vishnu and Shiva, represents the endless cycle of time

Brahman the ultimate ground of all being in Hinduism, the force or potentiality behind everything.

Brahmanas circa 800 to 500 BCE, commentaries on the four Vedas, expanded the systemization of sacrificial ritual

Brahmins the priestly and highest caste in India

Chakras energy vortexes (usually seven) where the prana gathers and spins, as its flow is concentrated where the main three rivers (nadis) cross. Muladhara (root), Swadisthana (sexual), Manipura (solar plexus), Anahatta (heart), Vissudhi (throat), Ajna (third eye) and Sahasrarara (crown) Chakra

Dharana concentration

Dharma duty, truth, vocation

Dhatus the seven basic bodily tissues or constituents of the human body

Doshas the three body-mind constitutions or biological humors in Ayurvedic, which are vata (air), pitta (fire-water), and kapha (earth-water)

Drishti fixed eye gaze

Dvaita "dual", traditions that believe enlightenment is brought about through a transformation in our essential state of being

Dyana absorption or meditation

Ekagrata one-pointed focus

Granthis "knots", hindrances or psychic blocks

Gunas basic characteristics of the manifest world. They are sattva, rajas, and tamas. The gunas always exist together and their interaction makes for the constant state of evolution of the universe

Hatha Yoga all physical practices of yoga

Hatha Yoga Pradipika "Light on Hatha Yoga". Contains a complete system of cleansing the body through six actions called the Shat Karma Kriyas

Ida Nadi the moon channel that starts in the left nostril and flows down to the right big toe

Ishvara "the Lord" or Supreme Being

Jiva Agni "fire of life" that lies at one's core behind the navel area

Jivanmukta one who is "liberated in life"

Jnana Yoga gathering wisdom from the study of the ancient scriptures

Kaivalya liberation

Karma "action", can be threefold: physical, mental, and somnial. All these actions will produce forces of retribution

Karma Yoga advocates the retributive benefits of rightful and charitable acts

Kriya a cleansing exercise

Kundalini (Shakti) the reservoir of psychic energy that lies dormant near our root, often represented as a three and a half coiled serpent goddess

Mandala "circle" or "completion", microcosmic pictures of the macrocosm of the universe. Meditations on mandalas are usually complex, involving contemplation on various symbolic meanings associated with different regions of the mandala

Mantra derived from the Sanskrit word manas, or mind, and the suffix -tra may denote a "getting beyond," a "tool" and "instrument", or simply to "liberate." A mantra refers to a sacred word or words whose sound vibration takes the chanter beyond the limits of his or her conditioned mind

Marma energy junctions, points in the body, which are used in martial arts, Ayurvedic massage and yoga practice

Maya-Leela the delusionary nature of reality

Meru Danda world axis

Moksha freedom

Mudra "seal", usually hand gestures, but some can involve other parts of or the entire body that fix an attitude and set a certain energetic circuit in the body

Nada Yoga the use of sound and deep listening to the inner resonance of the divine

Nadi "river" or "flow". Energy channels, along which prana flows. There are said to be 72,000 in the human body

Nirvana the cessation of suffering

Niyamas Observances, second Limb of Yoga

Padma Lotus

Panchamaya Kosha the five bodies or layers. These are the physical body (anamaya kosha), the vital body (pranamaya kosha), the mental body (manomaya kosha), the consciousness body (jnanamaya kosha), and the bliss-body (anandamaya kosha)

Pashupati god Shiva in his aspect as "lord of creatures"

Pingala Nadi the sun channel that starts in the right nostril and flows down to the left big toe

Prakriti "matter" or all that is not spirit. In Ayurveda denotes one's personal doshic distribution as determined at birth

Prana the vital life force, taken in primarily through the breath

Pranayama "restraint" and "harnessing" of vital life force, or prana. This is done through specific exercises in breath-control, which consist of inhalation (puraka), exhalation (rechaka), and retention (kumbhaka)

Pratyahara withdrawal of the senses

Purusha spirit

Quantum Physics applies the quantum theory to describe and predict the properties of a physical system

Rishis the seers who are said to have channelled the knowledge handed down through the Vedas

Saddhu, **Sannyasin**, **Sramana** ascetics

Sakshi the witness or ultimate observer

Samadhi enlightenment

Samkhya one of the oldest systems of philosophy in India and the worldview it presents is implicit in classical yoga philosophy

Samsara continuous and futile cycle of life and death, bondage

Sanskrit one of the most ancient Indo-Aryan languages, regarded as sacred in India

Sat-cit-ananda being-knowing-bliss

Shakti the feminine principle often associated with the generative force of nature. Also refers to energy and power

Shiva "the destroyer," the divine in its fierce aspect responsible for transcendental wisdom and yoga

Shruti "heard", implying a direct transmission of eternal truths

Siddhis supernatural powers

Smriti "remembered", derived from man's insight and experience

Sadhana spiritual practice

Spanda "pulse", which reflects the universal expansion and contraction

Sthira effort

Sublimatio "inviting awareness," or "fine-tuning" at the beginning of one's Quantum Yoga sequence. The term was originally taken from alchemy, and then applied in psychoanalysis

Sukha pleasure

Superimposition describes the fact that on a subatomic level, the building blocks of our material universe can exist both as particles and waveforms at the same time

Suryanamaskara Sun Salutations

Sushumna "ray of light" *nadi*, the central energy channel that runs along the spin

Tantra Yoga a later unorthodox development, which embraced the ecstasy of total sense immersion and the reversal of the flow of energy thus generated

Tapas spiritual fervor, the root "tap" denotes heat

Ujaii Pranayama "victorious breath". A lengthening, deepening and sharpening of the nasal breath through a contraction at the back of the throat

Upanishads (also referred to as Vedanta, or "end of the Vedas") about 1000 BCE. A new spiritual sentiment arises and with it a definite move away from ritual towards philosophy

Vayus the element air is categorised into five "winds", which represent the directional forces in the human body. Prana, Apana, Samana, Udana, Vyana

Vedas "knowledge". Collection of ritualistic formulas, chants, and pragmatic advice handed down in an oral tradition since ancient times. The earliest form of the Vedic canon, the Rigveda, dates at least as far back as 1500 BCE

Vinyasa "composition", breath-synchronized movement in a flowing dynamic yoga sequence

Vishnu "the sustainer," who keeps the cosmic order of the universe by manifesting in various forms on earth

Viveka skilful means and right knowledge

Yamas Restraints or abstentions, second Limb of Yoga

Yantras "support" or "instrument", visual tools for meditation made of basic geometric shapes

Yin-Yang taken from the Chinese cosmology and denotes the feminine, yin, as opposed to yang, the masculine principle

Yoga "union" with the Absolute, or "yoking" to the divine principle to realise ultimate truth and reach an enlightened state of consciousness

Yoga Sutras compiled second century BCE - third century CE by a prolific sage-scholar called Patanjali. The Yoga Sutras are divided into four padas, or chapters. Patanjali's comprehensive system is referred to as Raja Yoga, or the "royal path." Contains the Eight Limbs of Yoga, Ashtanga Yoga, which to this day form the basis for a yogi's way of life and practice

INDEX

Adho Mukha Svanasana, 60, 87-89, 98, 14, 116

Adho Mukha Vrikshasana, 51, 108-110, 112

Advaita Vedanta, 20, 87

Agni Sari, 78, 194

Ahimsa, 18, 35,

Amrit, 42-3, 138

Anusara Yoga, 24, 101

Archer (Dhanushmatasana), 90, 96

Asana, 26, 34, 103

Asceticism, 21-22

Ashtanga Vinyasa Yoga, 23, 66, 114, 229

Ashtavakrasana, 113, 202

Atman, 16, 43, 87, 212

Ayurveda, 47-55, 75

Baddha Konasana, 122, 138, 199, 203, 207

Badrasana, 148,

Bakasana, 111-112, 154

Balasana, 68, 82, 141, 146-7,

Bandha Triyam, 37, 53, 78, 81, 83-4, 108, 195, 218

Bandhas, 23, 34, 36-37, 42, 53-55, 61, 64, 75-81, 87-89, 98, 100-102, 106, 108-109, 114, 119, 123, 124, 128, 130, 136, 144, 156, 192, 206, 208-10, 217-8

Bhagavad Gita, 16, 21, 30

Bhakti, 10, 20-1, 23

Bharadvajasana, 207, 127,

Bhastrika, 53, 196-7

Bhekasana, 135, 137

Bhujangasana, 135, 137,

Bikram Yoga, 24

Bindu, 42, 105, 37, 219, 221

Brahma, 16, 20, 43, 87, 212, 216

Brahmanas, 16,

Brahmari, 200

Buddhism, 20, 72, 150, 156, 228

Chakras, 39-40, 43, 45, 74, 103, 117, 132, 136, 138, 141, 148, 194, 215

Chakrasana, 123

Chaturanga Dandasana (Chatwari), 60, 89, 114, 141

Dandasana, 118

Dhanurasana, 135, 137

Dharma, 13, 21, 125

Dhatus, 48-49

Doshas, 47-48 , 53, 64, 69, 72-73, 223-4

Drishti, 23, 88, 101, 106, 119, 136, 138, 216

Eka Pada Shirsasana, 123

Ekapadasana, 105, 109

Garudasana, 154

Golden Section/Ratio/Mean, 67

Gomukhasana, 124

Granthis, 42-43

Gunas, 28, 43, 47-48

Halasana, 138, 140, 143

Hanumanasana, 124, 218

Hatha Yoga Pradipika, 22, 42, 103, 212-4

Hatha Yoga, 63, 73, 100

Horse-riding Stance (Ashvarohinasana), 50, 68, 90-91, 96, 105, 109

Indus Valley Civilisation, 14-15, 35

Iyengar Yoga, 23, 66, 100

Janu Shirsasana, 117, 218-9

Japa, 215,

Jathara Parivartanasana, 136

Jiva Agni, 78, 90, 118

Jivamukti Yoga, 24, 230

Jnana, 11, 43

Kapalabhati, 194-5, 214

Kapha, 48-49, 51-55, 61, 69, 72-73, 98, 101, 119, 148, 156, 213, 223

Kapotasana, 134-5, 137, 154, 204, 216-7, 224

Karma, 10-11, 23, 28-29, 144

Kripalu Yoga, 24

Krishnamacharya (Shri Tirumalai), 23-24, 104

Kriya Yoga, 24

Kriyas, 22, 209, 212-4

Kumbhaka, 53, 78-79, 108, 192-201

Kundalini Yoga, 24

Kundalini, 40, 43, 45-46, 74, 80, 114, 156, 206

Lolasana, 114

Lutasana, 90, 96

Mandala, 156, 219-221

Mantra, 16, 24, 39-40, 47, 50, 54, 73, 90, 155, 215-6

Marichiasana 116,128

Marmas, 47, 75, 117

Matsyasana, 68, 136, 140-1, 143

Mudra, 24, 42-43, 75, 194-201, 212-4

Nada Yoga, 215-6

Nadi Shodana, 53, 192, 197-8

Nadis, 38-40, 73-74, 89, 100, 106, 121, 141, 144, 194

Nauli, 77, 79, 214

Navasana, 128, 131

Neti, 213

Padmasana, 121, 146-9, 156

Pancha Mahabhuta, 47

Panchamaya Kosha, 38-44

Parsvakonasana:

Utthita 98, 101-103, 105

Parivritta, 98, 105

Parsvottansana, 98, 105

Paryankasana, 124, 140, 143

Paschimottansana, 52, 119, 136, 208

Patanjali's Yoga Sutras, 10, 16-20, 25, 35, 87

Pavanmuktasana, 118

Pincha Mayurasana, 51, 108-110, 112

Pitta, 48, 50-55, 60, 69, 72-73, 86, 119, 144, 155, 200, 223

Prana, 38, 42-43, 48, 74, 81, 89, 100, 106, 121

Pranayama, 22, 26, 34, 42, 45-46, 52, 65, 73, 192-201

Prasarita Padottansana, 98, 105

Samadhi, 13, 17, 19, 22, 30, 84, 151, 216

Samakonasana, 124, 126

Samasthiti, 86

Samkhya, 16-17, 25

Sarvangasana, 123, 138, 140, 142-3, 204-6

Savasana, 40, 68, 141, 144, 146-7

Setu Bandha Sarvangasana, 135, 137

Shakti, 10, 20, 40

Shalabhasana, 135, 137

Shirsasana, 68, 123, 138, 141-3

Shiva Natarajasana, 64, 137, 204

Shiva, 10, 14-15, 20-22, 26, 40

Shivananda Yoga, 24

Siddhasana, 147-8

Siddhis, 22, 24-25, 27, 42

Sitali, 200

Spanda, 101-102, 116

Sukhasana, 147-8

Superimposition, 24

Suryanamskara, 24, 52, 60, 68, 86, 91-97, 103, 142

Tadasana, 52, 81-82, 84, 98, 109, 118

Tantra, 10, 51, 87

Tapas, 90, 155

Trataka, 213, 216

Trikonasana:

Utthita, 98, 100, 104, 105, 142

Parivritta, 98, 100, 105

Ujaii Pranayama, 23, 36-37, 64, 75, 80-81, 90, 123, 124, 128, 130, 140, 155, 193, 206, 209

Uncertainty Principle, 46

Upanishads, 16, 21, 67

Upavishta Konasana, 122, 138, 207-8

Urdhva Dhanurasana, 91, 134-5, 137, 203-4

Urdhva Mukha Svanasana, 60, 89, 114

Ushtrasana, 134-5, 137

Utpluthih, 144

Uttana Padasana, 140, 143

Vajrasana, 51, 82, 156

Vajra-vinyasa, 68

Vastu, 47, 219

Vata, 48-50, 52, 54-55, 60, 69, 72-73, 119, 130, 154, 223

Vayus, 41-42, 74, 206, 209

Vedas, 16, 21, 47, 104

Viloma, 53, 199, 203

Vinyasa, 23, 36-37, 60, 64, 72, 84, 90-91, 114, 116, 141, 154-6, 206

Viparita Karani, 205, 207

Virabhadrasana , 98, 102, 104, 105

Virasana, 51, 83, 123-124, 135, 146-8, 155

Vrikshasana, 106, 112

Vrischikasana, 110, 136-7

Yantra, 148, 219-221

BIBLIOGRAPHY

Al-Khalili, Jim, *Quantum: A Guide for the Perplexed*
(London: Weidenfeld & Nicolson, 2003)

Arewa, Caroline Shola, *Way of Chakras*
(London: Thorsons, 2001)

Bevan, Dr James, *A Pictorial Handbook of Anatomy &
Physiology* (London: Reed International Books, 1994)

Buddhananda, Swami, *Moola Bandha: The Master Key*
(Bihar: Yoga Publications Trust, 1996)

Burke, T.Patrick, *The Major Religions: An Introduction with texts*
(Oxford: Blackwell Publishers Ltd, 1996)

Choudhury, Bikram, *Bikram's Beginning Yoga Class*
(New York: Jeremy P.Tarcher/Putnam, 2000)

Coulter, H. David, *Anatomy of Hatha Yoga: A Manual for
Students, Teachers and Practitioners*
(Honesdale: Body and Breath, 2001)

Dean, Stanley R., *Psychiatry & Mysticism*
(Chicago: Nelson-Hall Inc, 1979)

De Michelis, Elizabeth, *A history of modern yoga*
(London: Continuum, 2004)

Feuerstein, Georg, *The Yoga Tradition: Its History, Literature,
Philosophy and Practice*
(Prescott, Arizona: Hohm Press, 2001)

Frawley, David, *Yoga & Ayurveda: Self-Healing and Self-
Realization* (Wisconsin: Lotus Press, 1999)

Frawley, Dr. David, Ranade, Dr. Subbash and Lele, Dr. Avinash,
Ayurveda and Marma Therapy: Energy Points in Yogic Healing
(Twin Lakes: Lotus Press, 2003)

Gannon, Sharon, and Life, David, *Jivamukti Yoga: Practices for
liberating body and soul*
(New York: The Ballantine Publishing Group, 2002)

Hartranft, Chip, *The Yoga-Sutra of Patanjali*
(Boston, Shambhala Classics, 2003)

Hawking, Stephen W., *A Brief History of Time*
(New York: Bantam Books, 1989)

Hinnells, John R. (ed), *A Handbook of Living Religions*
(London: Penguin Books, 1991)

Iyengar, B K S, *Astadala Yogamala*
(New Delhi: Alied Publishers Ltd, 2000)

Iyengar, B K S, *Light on Yoga*
(New Delhi: HarperCollins Publishers, 2002)

Iyengar, B K S, *Light on Pranayama*
(London: Unwin Paperbacks, 1983)

Johari, Harish, *Ayurvedic Massage: Traditional Indian
Techniques for Balancing Body and Mind*
(Rochester, Vermont: Healing Arts Press, 1996)

Jois, Sri K. Pattabhi, *Yoga Mala*
(New York: North Point Press/Farrar, Straus and Giroux, 2002)

Kapit, Wyn, and Elson, Lawrence M., *The Anatomy Colouring
Book – Third Edition* (Glenview: Pearson Education, 2002)

Lowitz, Leza, and Datta, Reema, *Sacred Sanskrit Words*
(Berkeley: Stone Bridge Press, 2005)

Mascaro, Juan, *The Upanishads: Translations from the Sanskrit*
(Middlesex: Penguin Books Ltd, 1974)

Miele, Lino, *Astanga Yoga – Second edition*
(Rome: Lino Miele, 1996)

Mishra, Ramamurti S., *The Textbook of Yoga Psychology*
(New York: Baba Bhagavandas Publication Trust, 1997)

Nagendra, Nagarathna, and Munro, Robin, *Yoga for common
ailments* (London: Gaia Books Limited, 1990)

Prabhavananda, Swami , *Patanjali Yoga Sutras*
(Mylapore: Sri Ramakrishna Math Printing Press, undated)

Rahula, Walpola, *What the Buddha Taught*
(New York: Grove Press, 1974)

Rieker, Hans-Ulrich, *Das klassische Yoga Lehrbuch Indiens*
(Zurich: Rascher-Verlag, 1957)

Roach, Geshe Michael, & McNally, Christie, *The Essential Yoga
Sutra: Ancient Wisdom for Your Yoga*
(New York: Doubleday, 2005)

Saraswati, Swami Satyananda , *Asana Pranayama Mudra
Bandha* (Bihar: Yoga Publications Trust, 2002)

Saraswati, Swami Satyananda, *Kundalini Tantra* (Bihar: Yoga Publications Trust, 2001)

Scaravelli, Vanda, *Awakening the Spine: The stress-free new yoga that works with the body to restore health, vitality and energy* (New York: HarperCollins Publishers, 1991)

The Sivananda Yoga Centre, *The New Book of Yoga – Revised Edition* (London: Ebury Press, 2000)

Svoboda, Robert E., *Aghora: At the Left Hand of God* (Bellingham: Sadhana Publishing, 1999)

Sweeney, Matthew, *Astanga Yoga As It Is* (The Yoga Temple, 2000)

Vasu, Rai Bahadur Srisa Chandra, *The Gheranda Samhita* (New Delhi: Munshiram Manoharlal Publishers, 2003)

Vyas, Bharti, *Simply Ayurveda* (London: Thorsons, 2000)

Ward, Keith, *Images of Eternity* (Oxford: Oneworld Publications Ltd, 1993)

Ward, Keith, *Religions & Revelation* (Oxford: Oxford University Press, 1994)

Wilber, Ken, *The Collected Works of Ken Wilber – Volume eight* (Boston: Shambhala, 2000)

Wilber, Ken (ed), *Quantum Questions: Mystical Writings of the World's greatest Physicists* (Boston: Shambhala, 2001)

Wood, Ernest, *Seven Schools of Yoga* (Wheaton: The Theosophical Publishing House, 1976)

Yogananda, Paramhansa, *Autobiography of a Yogi* (London: Rider and Company, 1980)

QUANTUM YOGA DVD

1. SPLASH SCREEN AND DISCLAIMER

2. MENU: TITLE PAGE

3. TRACK: INTRODUCTION

4. MENU: HEROES

Heroes: Regulating Pitta

Introduction

Sublimatio

Sublimatio

Viloma Pranayama

Supta Baddha Konasana

Utkatasana

Uttanasana

Tadasana

Ashvarohinasana

Bija Mantras

Dynamic Flow & Standing Poses

Dynamic Flow & Standing Poses

Tadasana & Bandhas

Suryanamaskara

Trikonasana

Parivritta Trikonasa

Parsvakonasana

Parivritta Parsvakonasana

Dhanushmatasana

Prasarita Padottanasana

Quantum Mini-Sequence

Bakasana

Samasthiti

Standing Balances

Standing Balances

Shiva Natarajasana

Floor Work

Floor Work

Triyanga Mukhaikapada Paschimottanasana

Kraunchasana

Bharadvajasana

Backbends

Backbends

Balabhujangasana

Ardha Bhekasana

Bhekasana

Chaturanga Dandasana

Urdhva Dhanurasana

Counter Pose and Core

Brahmandasana

Inversions

    Inversions

    Salamba Sarvangasana

    Halasana

    Parsva Karnapidasana

    Karnapidasana

Relaxation

    Relaxation

    Virasana Variations

    Supta Virasana

    Shavasana

Meditation

    Meditation

    Sukhasana

    Siddhasana

    Bhadrasana

    Virasana

    Metta Bhavana

Volker's Interview

    Volker's Interview

5. MENU: BIRDS

Birds: Regulating Vata

    Introduction

Sublimatio

    Sublimatio

    Tadasana

    Bandhas

Dynamic Flow

    Dynamic Flow, Vinyasa

    Suryanamaskara

    Ardha Kapotasana

    Adho Mukha Svanasana

    Uttanasana

    Virabhadrasana 1

    Virabhadrasana 2

    Pada Hastasana

    Samasthiti

    Malasana

    Bakasana

    Vasishtasana

    Bhujangasana

    Balasana

Standing Poses

> Standing Poses, Trikonasana
> Ardha Chandrasana
> Hip Alignment
> Parivritta Trikonasana
> Parsvakonasana
> Prasarita Padottanasana
> Samakonasana
> Hanumanasana
> Urdhva Mukha Svanasana

Standing Balances

> Standing Balances
> Vrikshasana
> Garudasana

Floor Work

> Floor Work
> Kapotasana
> Janu Shirsasana
> Ardha Matsyendrasana
> Gomukhasana
> Eka Pada Raja Kapotasana

Backbends

> Backbends, Shalabhasana
> Ushtrasana

> Baddha Konasana
> Upavishta Konasana

Abdominals

> Abdominals
> Upavishta Konasana
> Ubhaya Padangusthasana
> Navasana
> Navasana Variation

Inversions

> Inversions
> Halasana
> Karnapidasana
> Matsyasana
> Pavanmuktasana

Relaxation

> Relaxation, Shavasana
> Shavasana Adjustments
> Coming out of Shavasana

Meditation

> Meditation
> Mindfulness of Breathing

Tina's Interview

6. MENU: LOTUS-MANDALA

Lotus-Mandala: Regulating Kapha

Introduction

Sublimatio

Sublimatio
Balasana
Mula Bandha
Uddiyana Bandha
Vajrasana
Vajra Vinyasa
Marjara Variations
Adho Mukha Svanasana
Samasthiti
Tadasana

Dynamic Flow

Dynamic Flow
Suryanamaskara
Urdhva Hastasana
Dolphin

Standing Poses

Standing Poses
Ashvarohinasana
Prasarita Padottanasana
Parsvottanasana
Virabhadrasana 3

Arm Balances

Arm Balances
Pincha Mayurasana
Ardha Padma Vrischikasana
Vrischikasana
Adho Mukha Vrikshasana

Floor Work

Floor Work
Lutasana
Upavishta Konasana
Paryankasana
Half-Vinyasa
Ardha Baddha Padma Paschimottasana
Matsyendrasana

Abdominals

Abdominals
Urdhva Prasarita Padasana
Bharmanasana

Backbends

Backbends
Dhanurasana
Urdhva Dhanurasana
Supta Parivritta Garudasana
Chakrasana

Inversions

>Inversions
>Shirsasana
>Parivritta Pada Shirsasana
>Prasarita Kona Shirsasana

Relaxation

>Relaxation
>Sukhasana
>Padmasana, Yoga Mudra
>Kapalabhati with Jnyana Mudra
>Shavasana

Meditation

>Meditation
>Vipassana

David's Interview

7. MENU: BONUS MATERIAL

Sub-Menu: Pranayama

Pranayama

>Pranayama
>Preparation
>Agni Sari
>Kapalabhati & Bandha Triyam
>Bhastrika
>Nadi Shodana
>Anuloma

Menstrual Practice

>Menstrual Practice
>Supta Baddha Konasana
>Upavishta Konasana

Drishti

>Drishti

Avoiding Backpain

>Avoiding Backpain

Bija Mantras

>Bija Mantras

8. CREDITS

OTHER QUANTUM YOGA PRODUCTS

WWW.QUANTUMYOGA.CO.UK

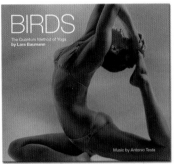

The underlying theme for Birds is freedom and is designed to remind us that yoga is a return to our natural state of ease and that all spiritual practice is ultimately a process of elimination leading us to the real self. Through practising asanas and vinyasa, we see the body return to its true shape, the nadis free up to allow for a harmonious flow of prana resulting in a deep sense of wellbeing. A safe and inspirational space is cultivated in which the body can express itself without the obstacles of the mind. Birds supplies a steady rhythm that supports the dynamic flow of a balanced yoga practice, in harmony with the breath. The sounds on this CD are produced from materials that possess the healing vibrations of natural sound, combined with the practice of yoga to create a positive energetic field in which true healing can take place. This double-album CD includes a fully comprehensive sequence chart of photographs. It is practiced in stages: at first CD 1 gives verbal instruction and music, supported by the visuals of the chart. Then CD 2 contains the same music that prompts one's memory; naturally the music can also be enjoyed in its own right. The final stage is to allow for variations and begin the act of true self-practice, inspired by the sequence of posture groupings listed at the back of the CD.

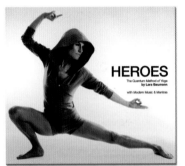

Yoga represents the methods and means that lead to a direct experience of the divine essence of reality. This sacred practice is approached with focus and discipline, referred to as tapas or spiritual fervour, whilst at the same time cultivating joy and encouraging playfulness. The body is purified through the heat generated from asana (postures) -vinyasa in conjunction with ujaii pranayama. The mind in turn is stilled and one's general disposition becomes cool and clear. A hero is neither aggressive nor reluctant to act, but instead masters the skill of balancing force with yielding. This sequence incorporates many variations on the hero's pose (Virasana) and is designed to smoothly strengthen every part of one's being. Thus it creates a steady platform from which to embrace our true form, realise our creative potential and bravely express our wild and loving nature. The word mantra is derived from man-"mind" and -tra "to cross over" or "liberate". On this double-album CD, these exalted phrases are repeatedly uttered in a musical way and the resulting vibration of healing sound, more even than their lyrical content, is said to carry transformative powers. A fully illustrated sequence chart is included.

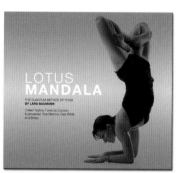

Yoga increases prana – the life force that brings vitality, health and happiness to the individual. Often through a sedentary life-style, a lack of inspiration and consumption of unhealthy foods, a person feels heavy, toxic and depressed. This means that a dynamic asana practice that maximises the aspect of vinyasa and incorporates invigorating, cleansing and stimulating postures should be developed. A Mandala in its basic form is a circle, which represents the spiralling upward motion that is encouraged in this sequence and echoes the mystical rising of kundalini shakti. It also symbolises a cosmic diagram, based on the sacred geometry of the macrocosm as reflected in the microcosm of the human body. We use this sacred geometry in yoga to re-align the body in such a way that allows an even and balanced flow of energy. Thus in the Lotus-Mandala, the strength and stamina inherent in the human organism in particular and the universe as a whole is drawn upon to realign itself with its true sublime shape. The artists who have contributed the music for this album use technology not to undermine or compete with natural sound, but rather to compliment and highlight its supreme beauty. Ill. chart incl. All net revenue from sales of this double-album CD go to the Usha Yoga charity. www.ushayogafoundation.org

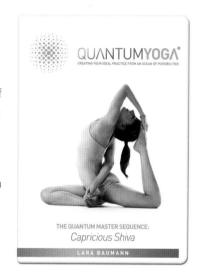

Capricious Shiva or the Quantum Master Sequence represents a challenging dynamic composition that brings the use of vinyasa to another level. Whilst always increasing prana or vitality, here the breath initiates, sustains and deepens movement, ensuring integrity and grace. The sequence includes strong core work, deep stretches, strengthening exercises and advanced arm balances. It encapsulates the essential qualities cultivated in all sadhana - an open heart, a strong core and an unwavering resolve to recognise what is false and undermining, and instead cultivate qualities that empower and illuminate. The DVD is accompanied by inspiring and beautiful music, which sets a positive mood and rhythmic pace. Experienced practitioners will be given the chance to further their understanding of vinyasa yoga, whilst integrating a creative system that leads to independent, intelligent and inspirational practice.